EMQs in Obstetrics and Gynaecology

Andrea Akkad
Consultant Obstetrician and Gynaecologist
Honorary Senior Lecturer in Medical and Social
Care Education
University of Leicester

Marwan Habiba
Senior Lecturer
Honorary Consultant in Obstetrics and Gynaecology
University of Leicester

Justin Konje
Professor in Obstetrics and Gynaecology
University of Leicester

Foreword by

David Taylor

Radcliffe Publishing
Oxford • Seattle

Radcliffe Publishing Ltd
18 Marcham Road
Abingdon
Oxon OX14 1AA
United Kingdom

www.radcliffe-oxford.com

Electronic catalogue and worldwide online ordering facility.

British Library Cataloguing in Publication Data

A catalogue record for this book is available from the British Library.

ISBN-10 1 84619 031 2
ISBN-13 978 1 84619 031 5

Typeset by Advance Typesetting Ltd, Oxford
Printed and bound by TJ International Ltd, Padstow, Cornwall

Contents

Foreword

Students determine the extent and depth of their learning by the type of assessment they will have to face at examination. During my time in academic clinical medicine, I have witnessed the evolution of undergraduate examination formats which I believe have gradually improved the quality of medical graduates. When I qualified assessment was by essay as a written format and the long clinical case as the clinical format. It came to be recognised that these were unreliable methods of assessing students' knowledge and clinical skills. Multiple choice examinations replaced the essay questions and became a more reliable format for testing knowledge, whilst different formats of the objective structured clinical examination replaced the long clinical case.

This book is, I believe, to be the first to assist students in obstetrics and gynaecology with a new format of testing knowledge and clinical skills, i.e. the extended matching question (EMQ). I am delighted my colleagues here in Leicester, where undergraduate education is given the very highest priority, have found the time and energy to write this book. This book comprehensively tests a whole range of obstetrics and gynaecology and I congratulate them for it.

Professor David J Taylor MD FRCOG
Vice Dean
Leicester Medical School
May 2006

Preface

Extended matching questions (EMQs) are increasingly being adopted as a format of written assessment, both in the undergraduate and postgraduate setting. EMQs have considerable advantages over formats such as multiple-choice questions (MCQs) and True/False questions, in that they test the application of knowledge and problem-solving in a clinical context rather than simple factual recall. EMQs appear to do so reliably, and there is less cueing and reliance on elimination of obviously incorrect answers. Consequently, it is likely that EMQs will replace many of the older written assessment formats. Many medical schools and professional bodies in the UK have either already introduced the EMQ format into their examinations or are in the process of generating question databases to be used in the not too distant future.

This book is intended to help medical students prepare for in-course assessment in obstetrics and gynaecology and final exams. Although it is primarily aimed at undergraduates, it will be also useful for specialist trainees in obstetrics and gynaecology who are preparing to take examinations at the postgraduate level by introducing them to the EMQ format. The standard of the EMQs included in this book ranges from easy to moderately difficult. However, both undergraduate and postgraduate readers should be aware that most question papers in high-stake exams are usually subjected to formal standard-setting procedures and the pass mark is therefore likely to reflect the difficulty of the paper, that is, the more difficult the paper the lower the pass mark. Our internal standard-setting process for EMQ papers puts the pass mark for undergraduates at between 50% and 62%, depending on the exact composition of an examination paper encompassing 40 stems. Naturally, postgraduates should be expected to answer the majority of these questions correctly. We hope that you find this book helpful in your course and exam preparation, and wish you the very best of success.

Andrea Akkad
Marwan Habiba
Justin Konje
May 2006

About the authors

Dr Andrea Akkad MD MRCOG is a consultant/lead for undergraduate education in obstetrics and gynaecology and honorary senior lecturer in medical and social care education at the University of Leicester and the University Hospitals of Leicester NHS Trust. Her main areas of interest in medical education are assessment and standard-setting. She is a keen question writer, and has recently led the successful conversion of the written undergraduate O&G exams in Leicester to an EMQ-based assessment format.

Mr Marwan Habiba MSC PhD FRCOG is a senior lecturer and honorary consultant in obstetrics and gynaecology at the University of Leicester. He obtained a PhD in medicine on endometrial responses to hormone replacement therapy (1998) and a PhD in ethics of health screening (2000). Mr Habiba pursues his research interest in the endometrium, healthcare delivery and ethics, and he leads a workshop on medical ethics for Leicester medical students.

Professor Justin Konje MD FMCOG (NIG) MRCOG holds a chair in obstetrics and gynaecology at the University of Leicester. His clinical and research interests include fetal growth disorders, recurrent miscarriage and endometriosis. Throughout his career Professor Konje has had a keen interest in medical education, and has contributed substantially to undergraduate obstetrics and gynaecology in Leicester. He has co-authored a number of books, including revision aids in obstetrics and gynaecology.

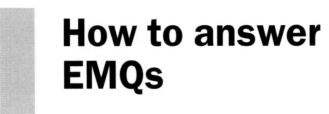

How to answer EMQs

EMQs consist of four elements: a theme; an option list; a lead-in; and a number of cases or stems. The *theme* is essentially the topic of the question, for example 'menstrual disorders'. The *option list* is a compilation of possible answers, which can consist of diagnoses, investigations, treatments, micro-organisms, anatomical structures and so on. The task to be performed in the question is specified by the *lead-in*, for example you may be asked to select the most appropriate diagnosis or investigation for each stem. It is usual for EMQ *stems* to be written in patient vignette format to give as much clinical context as possible. The level of assimilation required in the question may vary from stem to stem, so you may have a case scenario where the diagnosis is clearly given and your task is simply to select the best treatment option from the list; in more complex questions, the patient vignette may, for example, describe symptoms based on which you have to formulate a working diagnosis before you are able to select the most appropriate treatment.

Regardless of difficulty or complexity, the most useful approach to the EMQ is to read the lead-in (that is, select the most useful investigation) and the case scenario first. On reading the patient vignette, you should be able to answer the question *before* looking at the option list; when you do then read the options, you will be less distracted by other answers on the list. If the answer you thought of does not appear on the list, read the case scenario again to make sure you have not overlooked any important details.

It is not thought to be particularly useful in EMQs to go through the option list in an effort to eliminate incorrect answers. First, there may be a long list of answers (up to 20) and, second, when answering EMQs you are often selecting a best answer from a number of possibles rather than making a true/false judgement on each option. The patient vignette will contain clues to direct you to the best answer, so read it very carefully.

Although EMQs may vary in style and complexity, their basic structure, and the approach to answering them, remain the same. With a bit of practice, you should be able to answer questions in EMQ format successfully.

Reading list

Recommended reading

Greer I, Cameron J, Kitchener H *et al.* (2000) *Color Atlas and Text of Obstetrics and Gynecology.* Mosby, St Louis.

McCarthy A, Hunter B. (2003) *Obstetrics and Gynaecology. A Core Text with Self-assessment.* Churchill Livingstone, London.

Pitkin J, Peattie A, Magowan B. (2003) *Obstetrics and Gynaecology: an illustrated colour text.* Churchill Livingstone, London.

Symonds I, Baker P, Kean L. (2002) *Problem Orientated Obstetrics and Gynaecology.* Arnold, London.

Symonds EM, Symonds IM. (2004) *Essential Obstetrics and Gynaecology* (4e). Churchill Livingstone, London.

Reference books

Chamberlain G. (2001) *Turnbull's Obstetrics* (3e). Churchill Livingstone, London.

Drife J, Magowan B. (2004) *Clinical Obstetrics and Gynaecology.* WB Saunders, London.

Enkin M, Keirse M, Neilson J *et al.* (2000) *Guide to Effective Care in Pregnancy and Childbirth* (3e). Oxford University Press, Oxford.

James DK, Steer PJ, Weiner CP *et al.* (1999) *High Risk Pregnancies: Management Options.* WB Saunders, London.

Llewellyn-Jones D. (2000) *Fundamentals of Obstetrics and Gynecology* (7e). Mosby, St Louis.

Shaw R, Soutter WP, Stanton SL. (2002) *Gynaecology* (3e). Churchill Livingstone, London.

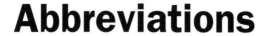

Abbreviations

AFP	alpha fetoprotein
BMI	body mass index
BP	blood pressure
COCP	combined oral contraceptive pill
CRP	C-reactive protein
CT	computed tomography
CTG	cardiotocography
DVT	deep vein thrombosis
FBC	full blood count
FSH	follicle-stimulating hormone
G	gravida
GI	gastrointestinal
GnRH	gonadotrophin-releasing hormone
Hb	haemoglobin
HCG	human chorionic gonadotropin
IDDM	insulin-dependent diabetes mellitus
IUCD	intrauterine contraceptive device
IUGR	intrauterine growth restriction
IUS	intrauterine system
LFT	liver function tests
LH	luteinising hormone
LMP	last menstrual period
MCH	mean corpuscular haemoglobin
MCV	mean corpuscular volume
MRI	magnetic resonance imaging
MSU	mid-stream specimen of urine
P	para
PCOS	polycystic ovary syndrome
PID	pelvic inflammatory disease
SHBQ	sex hormone binding globulin
STD	sexually transmitted disease
U&E	urea and electrolytes
UTI	urinary tract infection
WCC	white cell count

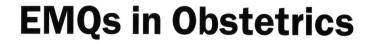

EMQs in Obstetrics

1
Normal pregnancy

Theme: Physiological changes in pregnancy

Options:

A   Increase in plasma fibrinogen
B   Reduction of renal threshold for glucose
C   Rise in cardiac output
D   Increase in red cell mass
E   Increase in creatinine clearance
F   Increase in plasma volume
G   Delayed gastric emptying
H   Inhibition of gonadotrophin secretion
I   Decrease in peripheral vascular resistance
J   Venous compression by enlarging uterus

Lead-in:

For each of the following case scenarios, please select the *relevant physiological mechanism* from the option list. Each option may be used once, more than once or not at all.

Q1   A 30-year-old G3 P2 presents for a routine ante-natal clinic visit at 22 weeks' gestation. She is very well and the pregnancy has been progressing in a satisfactory fashion. Her last recorded pre-pregnancy blood pressure was 138/85 mmHg. Today her BP is 88/50 mmHg.

Q2   A 23-year-old G1 P0 has a routine FBC taken at 36 weeks' gestation. This reveals an Hb of 10.0 g/dl (11.5–16.5), an MCV of 81 fl (80–90) and an MCH of 28 pg (27–32).

Q3   A 31-year-old G2 P1 presents for a routine ante-natal clinic visit at 32 weeks' gestation. Her blood pressure is 110/76 mmHg and the urinalysis reveals no protein, no nitrites and + of glucose.

Q4   A 22-year-old primigravida is admitted to the labour ward at 41 weeks' gestation in advanced labour; her cervix is 6 cm dilated and the fetal membranes are absent on vaginal examination. The fetal heart rate is satisfactory. She is given oral ranitidine by her attending midwife.

Q5   A 27-year-old primigravida at 36 weeks' gestation attends the ante-natal clinic for a routine appointment. She complains of vulval discomfort and on examination vulval varicosities are apparent.

Theme: Pregnancy milestones

Options:

A   20–22 weeks
B   9 weeks
C   6 weeks
D   16 weeks
E   34 weeks
F   12 weeks

G 3 days post-partum
H 42 weeks
I 36–38 weeks
J 12 hours post-partum

Lead-in:

For each of the following case scenarios, please select the *most likely time of onset* from the option list. Each option may be used once, more than once or not at all.

(Q6) A 33-year-old G3 P2, who has had two spontaneous vaginal deliveries at term previously, attends for routine ante-natal care in her third pregnancy. She has just started feeling fetal movements.

(Q7) A 23-year-old woman in her first pregnancy has undergone an emergency Caesarean section for delay in the first stage at 42 weeks' gestation. The baby was born in good condition. She is now feeling low, tired and tearful.

(Q8) A 29-year-old G2 P1 with an uncomplicated singleton pregnancy attends a routine ante-natal clinic appointment. Her symphysio-fundal height has been satisfactory so far. On examination today, the uterine fundus is palpable at the xiphisternum for the first time.

(Q9) A 38-year-old woman in her first pregnancy attends for routine ante-natal care. For the first time in this pregnancy, the midwife describes the presenting part as engaged.

(Q10) A 27-year-old G5 P3 with a viable singleton pregnancy attends for routine ante-natal care. The uterine fundus is palpable at the umbilicus.

2

Ante-natal care and pre-natal diagnosis

Theme: Ante-natal screening and diagnosis

Options:

A Amniocentesis
B Nuchal translucency screening
C Chorionic villous sampling
D Cordocentesis
E Fetal cardiac echo
F Pre-implantation diagnosis
G Sex selection
H Second trimester triple test
I Serum AFP
J Uterine artery Doppler

Lead-in:

For each of the case scenarios below, select the *most useful ante-natal test* from the option list. Each option may be used once, more than once or not at all.

(Q11) A 42-year-old G1 P0 seeks your advice about ante-natal screening and diagnosis. She is currently nine weeks pregnant. She would like to know whether or not her baby has Down's syndrome, and would like a test at the earliest possible opportunity.

(Q12) A 24-year-old woman with a 10-year history of IDDM presents for a booking visit at 22 weeks' gestation in her first pregnancy. Her HbA1c is found to be 10.1%.

(Q13) A 33-year-old G1 P0 attends for her booking visit at 11 weeks' gestation. She wishes to know the risk of her baby having Down's syndrome at the earliest possible stage.

(Q14) A 25-year-old G2 P1 attends for an ante-natal visit at 22 weeks' gestation. In her previous pregnancy she developed severe pre-eclampsia and intrauterine growth restriction, and had to be delivered by Caesarean section at 29 weeks' gestation.

(Q15) A 29-year-old woman presents for ante-natal counselling at 15 weeks' gestation. Her sister had a baby with Down's syndrome, and she would like to know whether or not her baby is affected.

Theme: Aneuploidy and genetic disorders

Options:

A   Edwards' syndrome
B   Turner's syndrome
C   Achondroplasia
D   Cystic fibrosis
E   Fragile X syndrome
F   Klinefelter's syndrome

G   Turner mosaic
H   Down's syndrome
I   Triploidy
J   Congenital adrenal hyperplasia

Lead-in:

For each of the case scenarios below, select the *most likely diagnosis* from the option list. Each option may be used once, more than once or not at all.

Q16   A 42-year-old G1 P0 declines the second-trimester Down's serum screening test, but attends for a detailed ultrasound scan at 21 weeks' gestation. On ultrasound the baby is small, has bilateral choroid plexus cysts and a 'rocker bottom' appearance of both feet.

Q17   A 24-year-old G2 P1 has a booking for ultrasound scan at 11 weeks' gestation, which reveals a cystic hygroma. She declines further testing and on subsequent scans the hygroma appears to resolve; she delivers a live female infant at 38 weeks' gestation. The baby has a webbed neck and bilateral pedal oedema.

Q18   A 39-year-old G4 P3 undergoes nuchal translucency screening at 11 weeks' gestation. This reveals an increased nuchal translucency, but the patient decides against invasive testing. At 21 weeks she undergoes a detailed ultrasound scan, which suggests the presence of a ventricular septum defect, a short femur, a thick nuchal fold and a sandal gap.

Q19   A 25-year-old G2 P1 undergoes a detailed ultrasound scan at 19 weeks' gestation. This reveals a significantly small baby and a disproportionately large placenta. The patient feels unwell during the scan and a midwife is called to see her. She finds her blood pressure to be 165/100 mmHg and there is +++ of proteinuria on urinalysis.

A 33-year-old G1 P0, who books late, undergoes an ultrasound scan at 28 weeks' gestation. This reveals a fetal head and abdominal circumference on the 50th centile, but all four limbs are below the 3rd centile. The sonographer also notes 'frontal bossing'. On further enquiry, the patient denies a history of musculoskeletal disorders in her or her partner's family.

Theme: Ante-natal risk assessment

Options:

A   Fetal growth restriction
B   Intrauterine fetal death
C   Macrosomia
D   Pulmonary hypoplasia
E   Trisomy 21
F   Congenital heart defect
G   Neural tube defect
H   Placenta percreta
I   Pre-eclampsia
J   Post-maturity

Lead-in:

For each of the case scenarios below, select the *most likely risk to the pregnancy* from the option list. Each option may be used once, more than once or not at all.

 A 29-year-old G5 P4, who has had four previous Caesarean sections, falls pregnant following contraceptive failure. The detailed fetal ultrasound at 22 weeks' gestation reports normal fetal anatomy and an anterior placenta which reaches the cervical os but does not cover it.

(Q22) A 37-year-old G1 P0 of Indo-Asian origin attends the ante-natal clinic at 35 weeks' gestation. She has no complaints, but you note from her hand-held record that her urinalysis has revealed glycosuria for the past three ante-natal visits.

(Q23) A 43-year-old woman is admitted to the labour ward with regular uterine tightenings, now occurring every three minutes. She is currently 27 weeks pregnant. She had an amniocentesis at 20 weeks' gestation because of soft markers for aneuploidy on her detailed anomaly ultrasound scan. The fetal karyotype was normal, but she reports that she has had a copious watery vaginal discharge since the amniocentesis.

(Q24) A 22-year-old woman books for ante-natal care at 19 weeks' gestation in her first pregnancy. She has epilepsy, and her seizures are controlled on sodium valproate 600 mg b.d.

(Q25) A 29-year-old G1 P0 attends the ante-natal clinic at 33 weeks' gestation, having had generalised pruritus for the past three weeks. It is becoming increasingly distressing and she has not been able to sleep properly for several nights. Her midwife took a number of blood tests two days ago and the serum bile acids are raised.

Theme: Teratogens

Options:

A   Lamotrigine
B   Warfarin
C   Ionising radiation
D   Rubella
E   Phenytoin
F   Cytomegalovirus
G   Varicella

H   Tetracycline
I   Vitamin A
J   Alcohol

Lead-in:

For each of the case scenarios below, select the *teratogen most likely to be responsible* from the option list. Each option may be used once, more than once or not at all.

(Q26)   A 26-year-old G1 P0 with a prosthetic mitral valve delivers a live male infant at 38 weeks' gestation. The child is subsequently found to have chondrodysplasia punctata.

(Q27)   A 31-year-old G3 P2 with epilepsy and gingival hyperplasia, who has not sought any ante-natal care, delivers a live female infant at approximately 34–35 weeks' gestation. The newborn has a cleft lip and palate, and a congenital heart defect.

(Q28)   A 31-year-old G2 P1 with spider naevi, palmar erythema and deranged liver function tests delivers a female infant at 33 weeks' gestation. The baby's birth weight is below the 3rd centile, and there is marked microcephaly and mid-face hypoplasia. The child is subsequently found to have moderate mental retardation.

(Q29)   A 19-year-old G2 P0 with a history of chlamydial PID delivers an appropriately grown baby at 41 weeks' gestation. In subsequent months, the child's teeth are noted to be of yellow-brown colour.

(Q30)   A 29-year-old G1 P0 delivers a live male infant at full term. Her pregnancy was uncomplicated apart from mild flu-like symptoms at 8–10 weeks' gestation. The baby has bilateral cataracts, sensorineural deafness, a cardiac malformation and microcephaly.

3

Common presentations in pregnancy

Theme: Early pregnancy

Options:

A Threatened miscarriage
B Ectopic pregnancy
C Retained products of conception
D Ruptured luteal cyst
E Urinary tract infection
F Complete miscarriage
G Appendicitis
H Incomplete miscarriage
I Molar pregnancy
J Missed miscarriage

Lead-in:

For each of the case scenarios below, select the *most likely diagnosis* from the option list. Each option may be used once, more than once or not at all.

(Q31) A 30-year-old woman in her fourth pregnancy attends for a routine ante-natal clinic visit at 16 weeks' gestation. She has had vague lower abdominal discomfort, but no bleeding per vaginam. She mentions that her nausea, breast tenderness and urinary frequency have now completely resolved. On examination her uterus is not palpable above the symphysis pubis.

(Q32) A 41-year-old P2 is 14 weeks pregnant by dates. Her periods were regular prior to pregnancy (5/35). She has had recurrent hospital admissions with excessive vomiting in this pregnancy, but has not yet had a dating ultrasound scan. At today's booking visit she is still complaining of vomiting, and the midwife finds the uterus to be large for dates on palpation.

(Q33) A 44-year-old G2 P0 calls out her midwife at 15 weeks' gestation. She reports a 24-hour history of spotting per vaginam, and is very anxious. She denies pain. The midwife finds her uterus palpable above the symphysis pubis and the fetal heart is audible with a SonicAid.

(Q34) A 39-year-old G3 P0 is admitted to the gynaecology ward at eight weeks' gestation. She reports a five-day history of spotting per vaginam. Over the past six hours she experienced increased bleeding with passage of clots and severe cramping pain. After passing a particularly large clot into the toilet, the symptoms of pain and bleeding appear to have resolved completely, but the patient is still anxious. On pelvic examination the uterus is of normal size and the cervical os is closed.

(Q35) A 22-year-old G1 P0 calls her midwife complaining of lower abdominal pain and vaginal bleeding. She underwent medical evacuation of the uterus three days ago because of a 'blighted ovum' at eight weeks' gestation. Since the intervention the bleeding has been getting progressively heavier and associated with intermittent cramping lower abdominal pain.

Theme: Abdominal pain 1

Options:

A   Urinary tract infection
B   Placental abruption
C   Red degeneration of fibroid
D   Musculoskeletal pain
E   Appendicitis
F   Pyelonephritis
G   Symphysis pubis dysfunction
H   Pre-term labour
I   Ovarian cyst torsion
J   Gastroenteritis

Lead-in:

For each of the following cases, please select the *most likely diagnosis* from the option list. Each option may be used once, more than once or not at all.

 A 25-year-old primigravida at 26 weeks' gestation is admitted to the labour ward with a one-day history of intermittent, sharp left iliac fossa (LIF) pain, associated with nausea. On examination there is marked tenderness in the LIF and features of peritonism. Her pulse is 100 bpm, BP is 122/67 mmHg and temperature is 37.0 °C. Urinalysis is negative.

 A 37-year-old G3 P2 of Afro-Caribbean origin presents to the labour ward at 32 weeks' gestation with severe constant left-sided abdominal pain. This is a singleton pregnancy. On examination the symphysio-fundal height is 36 cm. Her uterus is soft but irregular, and there is marked tenderness over the right side of the uterus. Maternal pulse is 114 bpm, BP is 119/62 mmHg and temperature is 36.9 °C. The fetal heart is 146 bpm. Urinalysis is negative.

(Q38) A 30-year-old primigravida at 28 weeks' gestation is admitted to the labour ward with a three-day history of abdominal pain and backache. The pain is worse on movement. She is currently in the process of decorating the nursery. On examination her uterus is soft, and there is mild generalised abdominal tenderness. Maternal pulse is 88 bpm, BP is 132/75 mmHg and temperature is 37.0 °C. The fetal heart is 142 bpm. Urinalysis is negative.

(Q39) A 17-year-old primigravida with a twin pregnancy at 20 weeks' gestation is admitted to the labour ward with a 24-hour history of worsening, right-sided, constant abdominal pain associated with nausea and anorexia. On examination her uterus is soft, but there is marked tenderness with rebound to the right of the umbilicus. Maternal pulse is 110 bpm, BP is 100/58 mmHg and temperature is 37.6 °C. The fetal heart rates are 168 and 159 bpm, respectively. Urinalysis is clear.

(Q40) A 41-year-old primigravida at 31 weeks' gestation is admitted to the labour ward with a six-hour history of intermittent abdominal pain and backache, which appears to increase in severity every 10 minutes. On examination the presentation is cephalic and the head is engaged. Maternal pulse is 100 bpm, BP is 122/67 mmHg and temperature is 37.2 °C; the fetal heart is 137 bpm. Urinalysis reveals + of protein.

Theme: Abdominal pain 2

Options:

A FBC
B Urine culture
C Blood cultures
D Abdominal X-ray
E Pelvic ultrasound scan

F MRI
G CT
H LFT
I Upper GI endoscopy
J Serum bile acids

Lead-in:

For each of the following cases, please select the *most useful investigation* from the option list. Each option may be used once, more than once or not at all.

(Q41) A 25-year-old primigravida at 18 weeks' gestation is admitted to the labour ward with a one-day history of intermittent, sharp left iliac fossa (LIF) pain, associated with nausea. On examination there is marked tenderness in the LIF and features of peritonism. Her pulse is 100 bpm, BP is 122/67 mmHg and temperature is 37.2 °C. Urinalysis is negative.

(Q42) A 41-year-old G3 P2 of African origin presents to the labour ward at 24 weeks' gestation with severe, constant, left-sided abdominal pain. On examination the symphysio-fundal height is 28 cm. Her uterus is soft but irregular, and there is marked tenderness over the right side of the uterus. Her pulse is 114 bpm, BP is 119/62 mmHg and temperature is 36.9 °C. The fetal heart rate is 146 bpm. Urinalysis is negative.

(Q43) A 38-year-old primigravida at 28 weeks' gestation is admitted to the labour ward with a three-day history of worsening upper abdominal pain associated with nausea and vomiting. On examination her uterus is soft, and there is marked tenderness in the right upper quadrant of the abdomen. Maternal pulse is 108 bpm, BP is 112/75 mmHg and her temperature is 37.5 °C. The fetal heart rate is 142 bpm. Urinalysis is negative.

A 17-year-old primigravida is admitted to the labour ward at 26 weeks' gestation with a 24-hour history of worsening, right-sided, constant abdominal pain associated with nausea and anorexia. On examination her uterus is soft, but there is marked tenderness with rebound to the right of the umbilicus. Maternal pulse is 110 bpm, BP is 100/58 mmHg and her temperature is 37.6 °C. The fetal heart rate is 159 bpm. Urinalysis is negative.

Q45 A 41-year-old primigravida at 28 weeks' gestation is admitted to the labour ward with a 12-hour history of intermittent abdominal pain and backache, which appears to increase in severity every 20 minutes. On examination the presentation is cephalic and the presenting part is free. The uterus is soft but irritable. Her pulse is 100 bpm, BP is 122/67 mmHg and temperature is 37.1 °C; the fetal heart rate is 137 bpm. Urinalysis reveals + of protein and ++ of leucocytes.

Theme: Anaemia

Options:

	Hb (g/dl) 11.5–16.5	Haematocrit (%) 37–47	MCV (fl) 80–90	MCH (pg) 27–32	WCC (×10⁹/l) 4–11	Platelets (×10⁹/l) 150–400
A	10.5	35	90	29	9	190
B	8.9	30	79	22	8.7	220
C	12.1	38	85	30	10	399
D	15.3	50	82	30	11	370
E	9.9	35	101	34	6	189
F	13.1	39	85	29	7.6	133
G	8.1	30	80	27	12.8	69
H	13.8	37	82	28	8.8	151
I	11.9	50	90	32	6.6	755
J	11.0	37	89	31	15.8	620

Lead-in:

For each patient described below, please select the *most likely full blood count result* from the options above. Each option can be used once, more than once or not at all.

 A 41-year-old G8 P5 presents for booking at approximately 29 weeks' gestation. She has a longstanding history of alcohol abuse and poor social circumstances.

 A 29-year-old primigravida is admitted from the ante-natal clinic at 30 weeks' gestation with a BP of 165/105 mmHg. She is complaining of nausea and vomiting, and of right upper quadrant discomfort. Her urinalysis reveals ++++ of proteinuria and + of blood.

(Q48) A 19-year-old primigravida of Indo-Asian origin presents for booking in at the ante-natal clinic. She has recently arrived in the country, and is thought to be approximately 11 weeks pregnant. You are taking a history via an interpreter. When asked about family history, the patient discloses that one of her siblings died in childhood from severe anaemia.

(Q49) A 30-year-old G3 P2, who has had hyperemesis gravidarum in both her previous pregnancies, is admitted at seven weeks' gestation to the gynaecology ward with excessive vomiting. She has not been able to tolerate any solids or fluids for the past week. Urinalysis reveals +++ of ketones.

(Q50) A 36-year-old woman delivers spontaneously at 33 weeks' gestation, having had pre-labour pre-term rupture of membranes from 29 weeks' gestation. She is re-admitted to the post-natal ward one week post-partum five days later with lower abdominal pain. On examination her temperature is 38.9 °C, pulse is 128 bpm and her uterine fundus is palpable at the level of the umbilicus and tender.

Theme: Shortness of breath

Options:

A Pulmonary oedema
B Pneumonia
C Pulmonary embolism
D Hyperventilation syndrome
E Physiological effect of pregnancy
F Pneumothorax
G Anaemia
H Heart failure
I Pleural effusion
J Asthma

Lead-in:

For each patient described below, please select the *most likely underlying cause* from the above option list. Each option can be used once, more than once or not at all.

(Q51) A 41-year-old G8 P6, who is currently 16 weeks pregnant, is admitted to A&E with acute breathlessness following a lengthy car journey. Her BMI is 38 and she smokes five cigarettes per day. She has no known medical problems. Her O_2 saturation in room air is 93%, pulse is 96 bpm, BP is 102/67 mmHg and her respiratory rate is 28 bpm. On auscultation her chest is clear, with normal air entry bilaterally.

(Q52) A 19-year-old nullipara with a BMI of 25 is admitted to the labour ward at 20 weeks' gestation complaining of chest tightness and breathlessness over the past two hours. She has no known medical problems apart from hay fever. On examination she appears dyspnoeic at rest and is using accessory muscles. Her O_2 saturation in room air is 95%, pulse is 122 bpm, and her BP is 102/67 mmHg. On auscultation there is widespread wheezing over both lungs.

(Q53) A 28-year-old primigravida with a BMI of 27 is admitted to the labour ward at 36 weeks' gestation complaining of occasional shortness of breath, fatigue, palpitations, dizziness and headaches. She has had symptoms for four weeks but only mentioned them to her midwife today. She looks pale, BP is 124/76 mmHg, her pulse is 104 bpm and her O_2 saturation in room air is 98%. Her chest is clear on auscultation.

(Q54) A 17-year-old GI PO, who is a known substance misuser, is admitted to hospital at 28 weeks' gestation with chest pain and breathlessness. On examination her BP is 100/66 mmHg, pulse is 104 bpm and O_2 saturation in room air is 95%. On chest auscultation she has right basal crepitations and there is bronchial breathing.

A 35-year-old GI PO is brought in by ambulance to the labour ward because of difficulty breathing for the past two hours. She is currently 24 weeks pregnant. She denies chest pain, but complains of dizziness and tingling in both hands; her symptoms started after she received some bad news about a member of her family. On examination her BP is 110/82 mmHg, pulse is 100 bpm and her O_2 saturation in room air is 98%. On auscultation her chest is clear.

Theme: Reduced fetal movements

Options:

A   Polyhydramnios
B   Maternal anxiety
C   Fetal dyskinesia syndrome
D   Anterior placenta
E   Fetal growth restriction
F   Placental abruption
G   Talipes equinovarus
H   Obstetric cholestasis
I   Drug effect
J   Vasa praevia

Lead-in:

For each patient described below, please select the *most likely cause for reduced fetal movements* from the above option list. Each option can be used once, more than once or not at all.

 A 41-year-old G6 P0, who is currently 18 weeks pregnant, is admitted to hospital having not felt the baby move for the past four hours. Her BP is 128/64 mmHg, pulse is 88 bpm, and urinalysis is negative. Her uterus is soft, non-tender, equivalent to dates in terms of size, and the fetal heart is heard with a SonicAid at 165 bpm.

(Q57) A 25-year-old G3 P2 is admitted to the labour ward with a
10-day history of reduced fetal movements. She is currently
32 weeks pregnant, and her dating and detailed ultrasound
scans were entirely normal. On examination her uterus is
tense but non-tender, and her symphysio-fundal height
is 37 cm. Her BP is 110/65 mmHg, pulse is 92 bpm and
urinalysis reveals +++ of glucose. A CTG is performed and
is found to be normal.

(Q58) A 28-year-old primigravida is admitted to the labour ward
at 34 weeks' gestation with reduced fetal movements for
24 hours. On examination her uterus is non-tender and her
symphisio-fundal height is 27 cm. BP is 154/96 mmHg, pulse
is 104 bpm and urinalysis reveals ++ of protein. A CTG is
performed and reveals a reduced baseline vari-ability and
absence of accelerations over a one-hour period.

(Q59) A 17-year-old G1 P0 is admitted to hospital at 28 weeks'
gestation with reduced fetal movements. She has been
feeling increasingly uncomfortable today. On examination
her uterus is tense and tender, and her symphysio-fundal
height is 32 cm. Her BP is 96/46 mmHg, pulse is 124 bpm
and urinalysis reveals + of protein. Auscultation with a
SonicAid reveals a fetal heart rate of 60 bpm.

(Q60) A 26-year-old G2 P1 is attending for a routine anomaly
scan at 21 weeks' gestation. She mentions that she is feeling
less fetal movements than she did in her last pregnancy.
During the ultrasound examination the fetal heart rate
appears normal, but only minimal movement is observed.
The sonographer is also concerned about the baby's posture
and the position of its limbs.

Theme: Vaginal bleeding

Options:

A   Placental abruption
B   Vaginal trauma
C   Vasa praevia
D   Vulvo-vaginitis
E   Placenta praevia
F   Cervical ectropion
G   Circumvallate placenta
H   Show
I   Cervical carcinoma
J   Foreign body

Lead-in:

For each of the following cases, please select the *most likely diagnosis* from the option list. Each option may be used once, more than once or not at all.

 A 25-year-old primigravida at 30 weeks' gestation is admitted to the labour ward with moderate fresh vaginal bleeding and abdominal pain, associated with irregular uterine tightenings. On examination her uterus is tender and irritable. Her blood pressure is 88/46 mmHg, pulse is 112 bpm and temperature is 36.9 °C.

 A 20-year-old primigravida at 38 weeks' gestation is admitted to the labour ward with fresh vaginal bleeding. Her membranes ruptured 20 minutes ago and she started bleeding immediately after they ruptured. On examination her uterus is soft, her pulse is 88 bpm, BP is 132/75 mmHg and temperature is 37.0 °C. The fetal heart rate is 90 bpm. Urinalysis is clear.

(Q63)   A 41-year-old G4 P2, who has had two previous Caesarean sections, is admitted to the labour ward at 32 weeks' gestation with sudden onset of heavy fresh vaginal bleeding. On examination her uterus is soft and non-tender. Her pulse is 120 bpm, BP is 98/52 mmHg and temperature is 36.6 °C. The fetal heart rate is 148 bpm. Urinalysis is clear.

(Q64)   A 37-year-old refugee of African origin, who is HIV-positive and has only recently arrived in the UK, books for ante-natal care at 22 weeks' gestation. She mentions a two-month history of heavy, fresh, post-coital bleeding following each episode of intercourse. On examination her uterus is soft and non-tender, and the fetal heart rate is 166 bpm.

(Q65)   A 22-year-old primigravida presents to the labour ward with vaginal bleeding at 17 weeks' gestation. She has had a thick, white vaginal discharge and vulval pruritus and soreness for the past week; for the past 24 hours she has observed blood on wiping herself.

4
Complications of pregnancy

Theme: Hypertensive disorders

Options:

A 24-hour urinary protein measurement
B FBC and coagulation profile
C Ultrasound scan
D 24-hour ambulatory BP measurement
E Urea and electrolytes
F LFT
G Uterine artery Doppler
H Renal ultrasound scan
I Chest X-ray
J MSU for culture and sensitivity

Lead-in:

For each of the following clinical situations, please select the *most useful investigation* from the option list. Each option may be used once, more than once or not at all.

Q66 A 42-year-old primigravida is undergoing induction of labour at 36 weeks because of hypertension and proteinuria from 31 weeks' gestation. She is on oral labetolol 200 mg tds. During the first stage of labour she becomes increasingly breathless and her O_2 saturations drop to 91–93%. You review her fluid balance chart and find that she is 2500 ml in positive balance.

Q67 You are asked to see a 25-year-old woman, 30 weeks into her first pregnancy, with a family history of pre-eclampsia, who was referred by her GP to the hospital with increasing pre-tibial oedema. She is asymptomatic. On admission her BP is 128/75 mmHg and her urine is clear. Symphysio-fundal height is 25 cm and the baby has been active.

Q68 A community midwife refers a 28-year-old P2 with two normal pregnancies in the past to the ante-natal clinic because of proteinuria. The patient is 24 weeks pregnant, and has made an appointment to see the midwife because of left-sided loin pain. On examination her BP is 125/60 mmHg, urinalysis reveals + proteinuria, +++ leucocytes, ++ nitrites.

Q69 A 23-year-old woman attends the ante-natal clinic at 22 weeks' gestation. In her previous pregnancy she developed severe early onset pre-eclampsia and fetal growth restriction, and had to be delivered by Caesarean section at 31 weeks' gestation. On examination her BP is 100/62 mmHg and her urinalysis is clear. Her detailed anomaly scan yesterday was reported as normal.

Q70 A 29-year-old G1 P0 with known pre-eclampsia is admitted to the labour ward in established labour at 37 weeks' gestation. She is on oral methyldopa 500 mg qds. She is requesting epidural analgesia.

Theme: Diabetes in pregnancy

Options:

A   Insulin regime and dietary modification
B   Metformin and dietary modification
C   Termination of pregnancy
D   Dietary intervention only
E   Induction of labour
F   Betamethasone
G   Caesarean section
H   Glibenclamide and dietary modification
I   Folic acid
J   Hypostop

Lead-in:

For each of the following clinical situations, please select the *most appropriate management* from the option list. Each option may be used once, more than once or not at all.

 A 36-year-old primigravida is referred by her midwife for a glucose tolerance test at 30 weeks' gestation because of a positive family history. Her fasting value is 6.2 mmol/l and the two-hour value is 9.1 mmol/l.

 A 28-year-old woman with pre-existing Type 1 diabetes is 38 weeks pregnant. Her blood sugar control has been satisfactory throughout the pregnancy, but an ultrasound scan at 37 weeks' gestation suggests an estimated fetal weight of 4.9 kg.

 A 44-year-old G4 P2 is referred for a glucose tolerance test at 27 weeks' gestation because of her BMI. Her fasting glucose is 8 mmol/l and her two-hour glucose level is 12.7 mmol/l.

A 30-year-old woman with recently diagnosed mild gestational diabetes, whose blood sugars have been satisfactory without drug therapy, is admitted to the labour ward at 29 weeks' gestation with painful tightenings. On examination she appears to be contracting every 20 minutes, and her cervix is effaced but not yet dilated. The baby is presenting by the vertex, and the fetal heart rate is satisfactory.

 A 32-year-old G3 P2 with well-controlled pre-existing Type 1 diabetes presents to the hospital at 37 weeks' gestation on two occasions with reduced fetal movements. According to a recent ultrasound scan, the estimated fetal weight is 3.35 kg and amniotic fluid volume is normal. Her first pregnancy resulted in a stillbirth at 39 weeks' gestation; the second baby was delivered by the vaginal route at 38 weeks' gestation.

Theme: Collapse

Options:

A Eclampsia
B Vasovagal attack
C Epilepsy
D Cerbrovascular accident
E Pulmonary embolus
F Postural hypotension
G Amniotic fluid embolism
H Cardiac dysrhythmia
I Hyperventilation syndrome
J Uterine inversion

Lead-in:

For each of the clinical presentations below, select the *most likely underlying cause* from the list of options. Each option may be used once, more than once or not at all.

(Q76)   A 21-year-old G1 P0 at 16 weeks' gestation is admitted to the hospital. She was out shopping with a friend; she suddenly felt faint whilst queuing at the till, became pale and sweaty and collapsed. The paramedics checked her blood pressure, and found it to be 96/52 mmHg, and her pulse was 90 bpm. Urinalysis is negative. She is now completely asymptomatic but is concerned about the baby.

(Q77)   A 29-year-old G2 P1 with gestational diabetes is induced at 39 weeks' gestation because of discomfort associated with polyhydramnios. She delivers spontaneously after a labour lasting only 45 minutes. A few minutes after the baby and placenta are delivered she suddenly collapses. Her BP is 70/35 mmHg, pulse is 146 bpm and thready, and she is cyanosed. You note that she appears to be bleeding from puncture sites on her arms.

(Q78)   A 39-year-old G1 P0 develops severe pre-eclampsia and labour is induced at 36 weeks' gestation. Her blood pressure is labile and difficult to control. You are called to see her when she complains of a headache. Her speech is slurred, and you find her blood pressure to be 238/160 mmHg. Urinalysis reveals ++ of protein. Whilst you are assessing her, the patient suddenly collapses and loses consciousness.

(Q79)   A 25-year-old primigravida, who is currently 29 weeks pregnant, is brought in by ambulance having collapsed at home. Her partner describes that she suddenly collapsed, her body went stiff and her limbs started to jerk. The attack lasted about two minutes. Her BP is 149/95 mmHg and her pulse is 88 bpm. Urinalysis reveals +++ of protein.

A 33-year-old G2 P1 labours spontaneously at term. She makes good progress in labour and delivers a live male infant. Syntometrine is administered in the third stage, but the midwife has difficulty delivering the placenta. She allows a further 15 minutes and applies controlled cord traction. The cord appears to be lengthening, but the patient suddenly complains of feeling unwell and collapses.

Theme: Obstetric haemorrhage

Options:

A   Rhesus antibody titre
B   MRI scan
C   CTG
D   Fetal blood sampling
E   Cervical smear
F   No investigation necessary
G   Ultrasound scan
H   MSU for culture and sensitivity
I   Apt test
J   Cordocentesis

Lead-in:

For each case scenario please select the *most useful investigation* from the option list. Each option can be used once, more than once or not at all.

 A 42-year-old G3 P2 who has had two previous Caesarean sections is admitted to the labour ward at 31 weeks' gestation with unprovoked, painless, fresh vaginal bleeding. The estimated blood loss is 150–200 ml. Fetal movements have been normal. Her vital signs are within normal limits, and the fetal heart rate is 145 bpm.

Q82 A 23-year-old primigravida, who smokes 20 cigarettes per day, is admitted to the labour ward at 29 weeks' gestation with fresh vaginal bleeding. She is also complaining of abdominal pain and reduced fetal movements. The estimated blood loss is approximately 100 ml. Her vital signs are within normal limits. At 20 weeks her placenta was reported to be fundal.

Q83 A 39-year-old woman who is HIV-positive attends the ante-natal clinic at 26 weeks' gestation. She complains of bloodstained vaginal discharge and recurrent painless post-coital bleeding for the past six weeks. Fetal movements have been normal.

Q84 A 26-year-old primigravida, who has had an uneventful pregnancy, telephones the hospital for advice. She is currently at 39 weeks' gestation and has had backache and irregular tightenings for the past 48 hours. The tightening has become more regular today, and she has noticed blood-stained mucus per vaginam on wiping herself. Fetal movements have been normal.

Q85 A 19-year-old primigravida who is Rhesus-negative attends for routine ante-natal care at 34 weeks' gestation. She has failed to attend her last two appointments, and has not seen her midwife since 22 weeks' gestation. A detailed ultrasound scan at 24 weeks' gestation did not reveal any abnormalities. She reports having had two episodes of painless vaginal bleeding at 25 and 26 weeks' gestation. Fetal movements have been normal, and her symphysio-fundal height is 36 cm.

Theme: Fetal growth disorders

Options:

A   Triploidy
B   Beckwith–Wiedeman syndrome
C   Gestational diabetes
D   Marijuana use
E   Obesity
F   Pre-eclampsia
G   Constitutional small-for-dates
H   Amphetamine use
I   Congenital cytomegalovirus
J   Antiphospholipid syndrome

Lead-in:

For each case scenario please select the *most likely cause* from the option list. Each option can be used once, more than once or not at all.

 A 30-year-old G1 P0 with a BMI of 24 is delivered by emergency Caesarean section for intrapartum fetal distress at 40 weeks' gestation. Her pregnancy is reported to have been uncomplicated. The baby's birth weight is 2.1 kg, and on examination, multiple petechial haemorrhages, jaundice and hepatosplenomegaly are noted.

 A homeless 20-year-old G1 P0 with a BMI of 18, who has only attended one ante-natal appointment during her pregnancy, is admitted with severe abdominal pain and vaginal bleeding at approximately 34 weeks' gestation. Her BP is 130/88 mmHg and urinalysis is negative. She is delivered by emergency Caesarean section and placental abruption is confirmed. The baby, whose birth weight is below the 3rd centile, appears jittery and irritable.

Q88   A 39-year-old G6 P1 with a BMI of 29, who has had four miscarriages in the past and a pulmonary embolism during her last pregnancy, is admitted to the labour ward with abdominal pain and vaginal bleeding at 35 weeks' gestation. Her BP is 128/88 mmHg and urinalysis is negative. She undergoes an emergency Caesarean section for suspected placental abruption. The baby's weight is below the 3rd centile, and the placenta is small with multiple thrombi and infarcts.

Q89   A 42-year-old G4 P3 with a BMI of 38 goes into spontaneous labour at 37 weeks' gestation. Her labour progresses well; however, the delivery is complicated by mild shoulder dystocia. The baby's birth weight is 4.8 kg. During the first 48 hours of life the baby experiences recurrent episodes of hypoglycaemia.

Q90   A 26-year-old G1 P0 of Indo-Asian origin with a BMI of 19 delivers spontaneously at 40 weeks' gestation. The baby, whose birth weight is on the 5th centile, is well and has an unremarkable neonatal course.

5

Therapeutics in pregnancy and puerperium

Theme: Drug therapy in pregnancy and puerperium

Options:

A   Methyldopa
B   Magnesium sulphate
C   Oxytocin
D   Warfarin
E   Dalteparin
F   Lamotrigine
G   Enalapril maleate
H   Sodium valproate
I   Syntometrine
J   Atenolol

Lead-in:

For each of the following patients, please select the *most appropriate drug therapy* from the option list. Each option may be used once, more than once or not at all.

(Q91)   A 19-year-old primigravida who is seven weeks pregnant attends the ante-natal clinic for a booking visit. She was diagnosed with epilepsy prior to pregnancy, but has not yet started treatment. She has had three grand mal seizures in the preceding week.

(Q92)   A 17-year-old primigravida is admitted to the labour ward at 36 weeks' gestation with a frontal headache and visual disturbances. She has had hypertension and proteinuria from 32 weeks' gestation, and her blood pressure has been controlled on oral labetalol. On examination she is hyper-reflexic and there is ankle clonus.

(Q93)   A 44-year-old G4 P3 is admitted to hospital at 36 weeks' gestation with sudden onset of chest pain. She is apyrexial, her O_2 saturations are 92–94% on air, respiratory rate is 26 bpm and pulse is 116 bpm.

(Q94)   A 39-year-old primigravida with a BMI of 38 is seen in the ante-natal clinic for a booking visit at 12 weeks' gestation. Her blood pressure is 145/92 mmHg and the urinalysis is negative. Two weeks later her BP is 158/95 mmHg.

(Q95)   A 28-year-old woman with aortic valvular stenosis (NYHA Class II) goes into labour at 39 weeks' gestation. She makes satisfactory progress and delivery is imminent. The midwife asks you to prescribe a uterotonic drug for active management of the third stage.

6

Labour, delivery and puerperium

Theme: Intrapartum assessment

Options:

A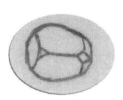

B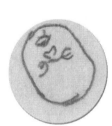

C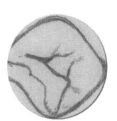

D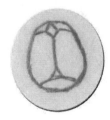

E

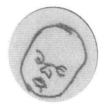

F

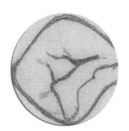

G

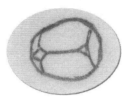

H

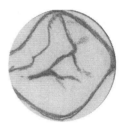

I

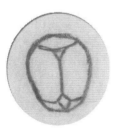

J

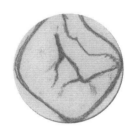

Lead-in:

For each case scenario below please select the *most likely finding on vaginal examination* from the options above. Each option can be used once, more than once or not at all.

(Q96) A 29-year old G2 P1 is admitted to the labour ward at 39 weeks' gestation with a four-hour history of painful contractions. The midwife examines her and finds a longitudinal lie with the presenting part fully engaged. On vaginal examination the cervix is 10 cm dilated and the presenting part is on the perineum.

(Q97) A 22-year old G2 P0 is admitted to the labour ward at 42 weeks' gestation in early labour, having ruptured her membranes 48 hours earlier. She makes very slow progress and her labour has to be augmented with oxytocin. She complains of severe backache throughout. The presenting part remains high, with 2/5 of the head palpable above the pelvic brim.

(Q98) A 39-year-old G6 P5 is admitted to the labour ward at 37 weeks' gestation in established labour. The midwife examines her and finds that her cervix is 7 cm dilated and the presenting part is very low, but finds it difficult to interpret her findings and suspects a breech presentation. A bedside ultrasound scan confirms a cephalic presentation but the head appears markedly deflexed. The patient delivers spontaneously within 30 minutes of admission.

(Q99) A 26-year-old G1 P0 undergoes induction of labour for hypertension at 37 weeks' gestation. There is delay in the second stage and a doctor is called to assess the patient. On abdominal palpation the fetal back is on the right and, after vaginal examination, the diagnosis of deep transverse arrest is made.

A 39-year-old G6 P5 is admitted to the labour ward at 42 weeks' gestation in established labour. On examination the midwife finds that her cervix is fully dilated and the presenting part is very low, but she suspects a breech presentation. A bedside ultrasound scan confirms a cephalic presentation but the head appears markedly deflexed. Delivery does not ensue over the coming hour despite frequent contractions and good maternal effort.

Theme: Management of labour

Options:

A   Immediate delivery by Caesarean section
B   Fetal scalp blood sampling
C   Oxytocin augmentation of labour
D   Subcutaneous terbutaline
E   Oral misoprostol
F   Intramuscular syntometrine
G   Instrumental delivery
H   Intravenous penicillin
I   Intravenous gentamicin
J   Repeat vaginal examination in four hours

Lead-in:

For each of the following patients, please select the *most appropriate intervention* from the option list. Each option may be used once, more than once or not at all.

 A 36-year-old G8 P6 arrives on the labour ward at 38 weeks' gestation, in established labour. On abdominal palpation the lie of the baby is transverse. On vaginal examination the cervix is 6 cm dilated and the membranes are bulging. Fetal heart rate is satisfactory.

A 19-year-old primigravida arrives on the labour ward at 42 weeks' gestation with regular painful contractions for the past four hours. On examination her cervix is 5 cm dilated and the station of the vertex is at the level of the ischial spines. Fetal heart rate is satisfactory.

 A 28-year-old G2 P1 is admitted to the labour ward at 39 weeks' gestation, in established labour. She is contracting every three minutes. Her cervix is 6 cm dilated, her membranes are absent and the station of the vertex is below the level of the ischial spines. The CTG reveals a fetal heart rate of 155 bpm with recurrent late decelerations.

 A 29-year-old G2 P1 undergoes induction of labour at 42 weeks' gestation for post-maturity. You are called to see her one hour after vaginal prostaglandin administration because of CTG abnormalities. You find that the CTG was satisfactory until 20 minutes ago, when the frequency of contractions increased to seven in every 10 minutes; over the past five minutes late decelerations have developed on the CTG. On examination the cervix is 1 cm dilated, 2 cm long and the presenting part is at –2 above the ischial spines.

 A 36-year-old G8 P6 arrives on the labour ward at 38 weeks' gestation, in established labour. Labour progresses quickly and the baby is delivered 40 minutes after admission. The patient wishes to have active management of the third stage.

Theme: Puerperal complications

Options:

A   Baby blues
B   Urinary tract infection
C   Thrombo-embolism

D Endometritis
E Breast abscess
F Post-natal depression
G Mastitis
H Post-partum thyroiditis
I Chest infection
J Puerperal psychosis

Lead-in:

For each of the following patients, please select the *most likely diagnosis* from the option list. Each option may be used once, more than once or not at all.

 A 30-year-old G5 P4 with a BMI of 38 undergoes an emergency Caesarean section in labour for fetal distress. On the third post-operative day the midwives become concerned as she appears to be mildly disoriented. She is not on any medication except oral analgesia. Her temperature is 37.3 °C, respiratory rate is 24 bpm and pulse is 114 bpm. Her jugular venous pressure (JVP) is raised and O_2 saturation is 91% in room air, but her chest is clear on auscultation. Her wound appears to be healing well, her uterus is well involuted and non-tender and her urinalysis is negative.

 A 29-year-old single G1 P0 undergoes an emergency Caesarean section after a prolonged labour. She is discharged home on the third post-operative day, although there is some concern about her mood. The community midwife visits daily; on day 5 she finds the patient confused, disoriented and complaining of hearing voices. She is apyrexial, with normal observations and her urinalysis is negative. The uterus is adequately involuted and her lochia is normal.

Q108 A 17-year-old G1 P0 undergoes an emergency Caesarean section after a prolonged labour and a failed attempt at instrumental delivery. On the third post-operative day she appears unwell and complains of lower abdominal pain. On examination her temperature is 37.9 °C and pulse is 104 bpm. Her uterus is palpable at the umbilicus and tender. The wound is healing well. On inspection of her pad, the lochia appears heavy and offensive. Urinalysis reveals + of protein and ++ of ketones.

Q109 A 38-year-old G1 P0 undergoes an elective Caesarean section for breech presentation. On the fourth post-operative day she complains of lower abdominal pain. On examination her temperature is 37.1 °C and her pulse is 88 bpm. Her uterus is non-tender and just palpable above the symphysis pubis; her lochia is normal. The wound is healing well, but there is marked suprapubic tenderness. Urinalysis reveals + of protein and ++ of nitrites.

Q110 A 25-year-old G1 P0 undergoes an emergency Caesarean section after a prolonged labour. On the third post-operative day she appears unwell, her temperature is 37.5 °C and pulse is 100 bpm. Urinalysis reveals + of blood. The midwife asks you to assess the patient. On examination her uterus is non-tender and just palpable above the symphysis pubis and her lochia is normal. The wound is healing well. She has some bilateral breast tenderness, but there is erythema and marked tenderness in the left breast. The area is not fluctuant.

EMQs in
Gynaecology

7

Anatomy and sexual differentiation

Theme: Pelvic anatomy

Options:

A   Round ligament
B   Falciform ligament
C   Sacrospinous ligament
D   Broad ligament
E   Pectineal ligament
F   Uterosacral ligament
G   Umbilical ligament
H   Infundibulo-pelvic ligament
I   Ovarian ligament
J   Lateral arcuate ligament

Lead-in:

For each description below, please select the *correct anatomical structure* from the option list. Each option may be used once, more than once or not at all.

(Q111) A 30-year-old woman undergoes an abdominal hysterectomy with conservation of ovaries. The surgeon divides the structure connecting the ovaries to the uterus.

(Q112) A 39-year-old woman undergoes laparoscopic sterilisation by Filshie clips. She falls pregnant six months later, and subsequently it transpires that the surgeon had mistakenly placed the clips on the structures anterior to the Fallopian tubes.

(Q113) A 45-year-old woman undergoes a total abdominal hysterectomy and bilateral salpingo-oophorectomy. The surgeon divides the structure containing the ovarian vessels.

(Q114) A 33-year-old woman presents with dysmenorrhoea and deep dyspareunia. On vaginal examination there is a tender nodularity palpable through the posterior vaginal fornix.

(Q115) A 35-year-old woman is diagnosed with cervical carcinoma. On vaginal examination there is bilateral induration lateral to the cervix.

Theme: Sexual differentiation and development

Options:

A   46 XX
B   45 XO
C   47 XYY
D   47 XXY
E   47 XY +21
F   47 XX +18
G   48 XXXY
H   46 XY

I   47 XX +13
J   46 XY/45 X0 mosaic

Lead-in:

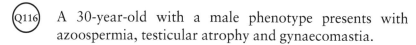

For each of the following clinical conditions, please select the *most likely karyotype* from the option list. Each option may be used once, more than once or not at all.

Q116   A 30-year-old with a male phenotype presents with azoospermia, testicular atrophy and gynaecomastia.

Q117   A phenotypically female 22-year-old presents with primary amenorrhoea, short stature, shield thorax and aortic co-arctation.

Q118   A 14-year-old child with a female phenotype enters puberty and virilisation occurs. Following investigations, 5-alpha-reductase deficiency is diagnosed.

Q119   A phenotypically female 17-year-old presents with primary amenorrhoea; assessment reveals normal secondary sexual characteristics, normal female gonads and an absent uterus.

Q120   A 27-year-old with a female phenotype presents with secondary amenorrhoea of 18 months' duration and a negative pregnancy test. She is of average height and weight with normal secondary sexual characteristics; her history includes two terminations of pregnancy as a teenager.

8

Sexual health and family planning

Theme: Female genital tract infections

Options:

A *Chlamydia trachomatis*
B *Herpes simplex* virus
C *Gardnerella vaginalis*
D Group B haemolytic streptococcus
E *Candida albicans*
F *Chlamydia psittaci*
G Human papilloma virus
H *Trichomonas vaginalis*
I Döderline bacilli
J *Yersinia pestis*

Lead-in:

For each of the following clinical presentations, please select the *organism most likely to be responsible* from the option list. Each option may be used once, more than once or not at all.

Q121 A 21-year-old woman is admitted to hospital with severe vulval pain and inability to pass urine for the preceding 24 hours. On examination she has significant bilateral labial oedema and multiple small, ulcerated lesions on both labia minora.

Q122 A 21-year-old nulliparous woman, who had an ectopic pregnancy six months ago, is admitted to hospital with acute lower abdominal pain and mild pyrexia. She has lower abdominal tenderness, positive cervical excitation and bilateral adnexal tenderness. On speculum examination there is copious muco-purulent cervical discharge. Her pregnancy test is negative.

Q123 A 17-year-old girl attends her GP's surgery complaining of 'lumps' down below. On inspection, there are multiple non-tender vulval and perineal whitish papular lesions with areas of keratinisation.

Q124 A 30-year-old woman, who is 12 weeks pregnant, complains of vaginal discharge. A culture of a mid-stream specimen of urine, taken routinely at her booking visit 10 days previously, revealed Gram-positive cocci. Her last baby suffered severe neonatal sepsis, and spent the first two post-natal weeks in the neonatal intensive care unit.

Q125 A 39-year-old woman complains of an offensive and irritant vaginal discharge. On examination there is vulval and vaginal erythema, and vulval excoriations. On speculum examination there is a copious grey discharge.

Theme: Family planning

Options:

A   Female sterilisation
B   Combined oral contraceptive pill
C   Depot-Provera
D   Male sterilisation
E   Progestogen-only pill
F   Levonorgestrel intrauterine system
G   Intrauterine contraceptive device
H   Levonelle
I   Male condom
J   Mifepristone

Lead-in:

For each of the patients described below, please recommend the *most appropriate contraceptive method* from the option list. Each option may be used once, more than once or not at all.

 A 24-year-old woman presents to the family planning clinic on day 16 of her current cycle, having had unprotected intercourse on days 11, 13 and 14. She is nulliparous and her cycles are regular at 4/28.

 A 35-year-old parous woman, who is on antihypertensive medication and has a BMI of 40, consults her GP about contraception. She and her partner are currently using condoms for contraception, but she would prefer a longer-term method that does not require particular attention to compliance. She is considering female sterilisation. Her periods are regular but heavy, with passage of clots and flooding, causing her to miss work and social engagements occasionally.

Q128 A 16-year-old schoolgirl with irregular, heavy and painful periods requests reliable contraception following a condom mishap.

Q129 A 23-year-old nulliparous woman attends her GP's surgery for contraceptive advice. She is about to join an aid agency and will be posted to a developing country with poor access to medical services for the coming 12 months. She would like a long-acting, reversible method of contraception.

Q130 A 43-year-old nulliparous woman asks you for contraceptive advice; she would like a contraceptive with a high efficacy because of her medical history. She is hypertensive and is fully anticoagulated because of recurrent pulmonary embolism. Her periods are regular and light with a cycle of 3/35, and she does not wish to use a contraceptive that would affect her menstrual cycle. Several attempts have been made to site an IUCD, but these have failed because of a stenosed cervical os. Her 49-year-old partner, who is very supportive, has four children from a previous marriage.

9

Physiology and pathology of the menstrual cycle

Theme: Physiology of menstruation

Options:

A Progesterone
B Oestradiol
C Follicle-stimulating hormone
D Sex hormone binding globulin
E Luteinising hormone
F Oestriol
G Inhibin
H Relaxin
I Androstenedione
J Dehydroepiandrosterone

Lead-in:

For each of the following scenarios, please select the *hormone most likely to be responsible* from the option list. Each option may be used once, more than once or not at all.

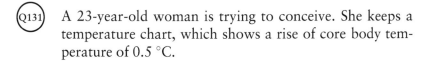

Q131   A 23-year-old woman is trying to conceive. She keeps a temperature chart, which shows a rise of core body temperature of 0.5 °C.

Q132   A 27-year-old nulliparous woman is undergoing investigations for infertility. Her doctor wishes to perform a blood test to confirm ovulation.

Q133   A 30-year-old woman with a regular menstrual cycle is trying to conceive. She buys an 'ovulation prediction' kit from her local chemist, which requires her to perform urine testing for five consecutive days each cycle.

Q134   A 29-year-old nulliparous woman, who is not using any contraception, attends for a cervical smear. On speculum examination she is noted to have copious clear cervical mucus, which shows *spinnbarkeit*.

Q135   A 36-year-old woman experiences breast tenderness, bloating and lethargy in the week coming up to menstruation.

Theme: Histopathology of the endometrium

Options:

A   Proliferative endometrium
B   Adenocarcinoma
C   Atrophic endometrium
D   Simple hyperplasia
E   Secretory endometrium
F   Decidua
G   Luteal phase defect
H   Complex hyperplasia
I   Squamous cell carcinoma
J   Atypical hyperplasia

Lead-in:

For each of the following clinical presentations, please select the *most likely histopathological diagnosis* from the option list. Each option may be used once, more than once or not at all.

(Q136) A 50-year-old woman attends the gynaecology clinic because of heavy periods whilst taking cyclical combined HRT. An endometrial biopsy is taken on day 23 of the HRT pack, and is sent for histopathological assessment.

(Q137) A 38-year-old woman undergoes a laparoscopy for suspected ectopic pregnancy. The surgeon suspects a tubal abortion has taken place. The patient's uterine cavity is curetted and the curettings are sent for histopathological assessment.

(Q138) A 66-year-old healthy parous woman with a BMI of 26 presents following a single episode of post-menopausal bleeding. Ultrasound suggests an endometrial thickness of 3 mm. An endometrial biopsy is taken and sent for histopathological assessment.

(Q139) A 66-year-old nulliparous woman with a BMI of 41 presents with recurrent post-menopausal bleeding. Her medical history includes hypertension and diabetes mellitus. Ultrasound suggests irregular endometrium with a thickness of 10 mm. An endometrial biopsy is taken and sent for histopathological assessment.

(Q140) A 41-year-old woman, who was sterilised 12 months ago, attends the gynaecology clinic with regular heavy periods. Her cycles are 5/28, but for the past year they have become increasingly heavy and she occasionally has to wear double sanitary protection. Her work and social life have not been affected. Her LMP was 10 days ago. An endometrial biopsy is taken and sent for histopathological assessment.

Theme: Menstrual disorders

Options:

A   CT scan
B   Diagnostic laparoscopy
C   Endometrial biopsy
D   Thyroid function test
E   APTT and platelet function tests
F   Pelvic ultrasound
G   Serum FSH, LH
H   High vaginal swab
I   Thrombophilia screen
J   Cervical smear

Lead-in:

For each of the following clinical presentations, please select the *most appropriate first-line investigation* from the option list. Each option may be used once, more than once or not at all.

 A 48-year-old woman attends the gynaecology clinic with heavy irregular periods. Her menstrual loss is associated with passage of clots and flooding. There are no other associated symptoms. She has been on ferrous sulphate tablets for the last six weeks and her recent Hb was 11.1 g/dl. Examination reveals a normal-sized uterus and normal adnexa.

 A 38-year-old woman with a BMI of 41 attends the gynaecology clinic. She was sterilised three years ago and since then has been complaining of heavy periods. She bleeds for seven days every month, and experiences passage of clots and flooding for the first 3–4 days of her period. She has been on ferrous sulphate tablets for the last six weeks and her Hb has increased from 9.4 g/dl to 11.5 g/dl. On pelvic examination she is markedly tender in the left iliac fossa.

Q143 A 36-year-old P1 presents with a one-year history of light infrequent periods, which can be up to eight months apart. She bleeds for one or two days in the form of spotting. Recently, she has been complaining of headaches. She has no hirsutism or galactorrhoea. Her BMI is 22. Physical examination does not reveal any abnormalities. Her GP had requested a serum prolactin level, which was 1107 pmol/l (50–400).

Q144 A 33-year-old G3 P3 attends the gynaecology clinic with heavy regular periods. She discontinued the combined oral contraceptive pill (COCP) four years ago because of the pill scare and her husband has since had a vasectomy. She would like to restart the COCP as it controlled her periods very well, but her GP is reluctant to prescribe it as her sister suffered a DVT following a Caesarean section.

Q145 A 43-year-old woman, who has regular light periods, attends the gynaecology clinic with post-coital bleeding. She also mentions several episodes of intermenstrual spotting. Her recent Hb was 12.1 g/dl.

Theme: Amenorrhoea/ oligomenorrhoea

Options:

	FSH (1–20) iU/l	LH (1–20) iU/l	Oestradiol (130–1500) pmol/l	Testoster-one (0.2–3.0) nmol/l	Sex hormone binding globulin (30–75) nmol/l	Prolactin (50–500) mU/l
A	60	55	<70	3.0	28	159
B	3	15	150	3.3	15	220
C	7	4	355	0.9	63	172
D	<1	<1	80	0.2	88	33
E	6	11	788	0.7	30	189
F	6.5	3	135	2.5	33	1420
G	12	5.9	265	1.1	56	500
H	13	5	550	2.0	70	151
I	8	4.2	129	0.8	65	499
J	6	11	300	2.9	40	405

Lead-in:

For each of the clinical case scenarios below, select the *most likely follicular phase endocrine profile* from the table above. Each option may be used once, more than once or not at all.

 A 30-year-old woman presents with secondary amenorrhoea of eight months' duration and galactorrhoea. She is not using contraception, but her pregnancy test is negative.

(Q147) A 45-year-old woman presents with secondary amenorrhoea for the past six months, vaginal dryness and reduced libido. She uses condoms for contraception. Her pregnancy test is negative.

(Q148) A 20-year-old woman presents with amenorrhoea of one year's duration. This was preceded by significant weight loss, and her BMI is now 15. Her pregnancy test is negative.

(Q149) A 29-year-old woman presents with oligomenorrhoea and acne. Her weight has progressively increased over the past two years, and her BMI is now 37. A pregnancy test is negative.

(Q150) A 31-year-old woman presents with a 12-month history of amenorrhoea, headaches and visual field defects. Her pregnancy test is negative.

10

Infertility

Theme: Investigating infertile couples

Options:

A Hysteroscopy
B Semen analysis
C Serum follicle-stimulating hormone
D Day 21 progesterone
E Free androgen index
F High vaginal swab
G Laparoscopy and dye pertubation
H FBC
I Rubella antibody titre
J Serum prolactin

Lead-in:

For each of the following clinical presentations of infertile couples, please select the *single most useful investigation* from the option list. Each option may be used once, more than once or not at all.

 Q151 A 29-year-old woman presents with a three-year history of primary infertility. Her menstrual cycles are regular at 5/28, and she denies pelvic pain or dyspareunia. She had chickenpox as a child, but otherwise there is no significant past medical or gynaecological history. Her partner is also fit and well, and gives a history of the usual childhood diseases, including measles, mumps and chickenpox.

Q152   A 35-year-old woman presents with a two-year history of secondary infertility. She had a successful pregnancy three years ago with the same partner. She had a normal vaginal delivery at term, but underwent surgical evacuation of the uterus two weeks post-partum because of suspected retained products of conception. Her menstrual cycle has been regular since at 1/29, but very light, amounting to spotting only. Her partner is fit and well.

Q153   A 32-year-old woman, who has cycles of 7/28 with heavy and painful periods, presents with a one-year history of secondary infertility. She had a successful pregnancy six years ago. She used an IUCD subsequently, which had to be removed because of lower abdominal pain and offensive discharge. Her partner of two years has three children from two previous relationships.

Q154   A 29-year-old woman presents with a one-year history of secondary infertility. Her cycles are usually 3/31, but she has been amenorrhoeic for 14 months. Her pregnancy test is negative. Her first child was born by normal vaginal delivery 18 months ago. She went on to develop puerperal psychosis and has been on anti-psychotic medication since.

Q155   A 21-year-old woman presents to her GP anxious about her inability to conceive. She is fit and well, and her menstrual cycle is regular at 3/26, with no pathological features. Her partner of six months is also healthy, and has a child from a previous relationship. She has been trying to conceive for the past three months.

Theme: Causes of infertility

Options:

A   Tubal disease
B   Endometriosis
C   Anovulation
D   Pituitary microadenoma
E   Klinefelter's syndrome
F   Testicular feminisation
G   Antisperm antibodies
H   Lifestyle factors
I   Uterine fibroids
J   Asherman's syndrome
K   Congenital uterine malformation

Lead-in:

For each of the following clinical presentations of infertile couples, please select the *most likely diagnosis* from the option list. Each option may be used once, more than once or not at all.

 One-year history of secondary infertility in a 32-year-old woman, who has regular cycles of 7/28. Her periods are heavy and painful. She had a successful pregnancy six years ago. She used an IUCD subsequently, which had to be removed because of lower abdominal pain and offensive vaginal discharge. Her partner of two years has three children from two previous relationships.

 Two-year history of primary infertility in a 35-year-old nulliparous woman with cycles 4/26. Her periods are not unduly heavy, but, since she has discontinued the combined oral contraceptive pill in order to conceive, they have been painful to the extent that she misses work. Her partner comments that intercourse is infrequent because she finds it too uncomfortable.

Q158 Three-year history of primary infertility in a 25-year-old woman with cycles of 8/45–80. Her BMI is 38. Her partner, who is 30 years old, is fit and well.

Q159 Two-year history of secondary infertility in a 29-year-old housewife. Her cycles are usually regular at 3/32; there is no history of gynaecological disorders or any significant medical history. Her partner is also healthy; however, because of his work commitments they spend almost six months of each year apart.

Q160 Two-year history of secondary infertility in a 35-year-old woman with cycles of 6/29. There is no significant medical or gynaecological history. Her partner had a vasectomy six years ago, which was reversed two years ago.

11

Common gynaecological presentations

Theme: Urinary symptoms

Options:

A   Urethral diverticulum
B   Urodynamic (genuine) stress incontinence
C   Detrusor instability
D   Overflow incontinence
E   Vesico-vaginal fistula
F   Carcinoma of the bladder
G   Urinary tract infection
H   Neurogenic bladder
I   Urogenital atrophy
J   Interstitial cystitis

Lead-in:

For each of the clinical case scenarios below, select the *most likely diagnosis* from the list of options. Each option may be used once, more than once or not at all.

Q161 A 49-year-old woman complains of frequency, urgency and nocturia. Her input–output chart shows that she drinks eight cups of coffee per day, but the intake volumes are not excessive. She voids in approximately two-hourly intervals during daytime, with a maximum voiding volume of 100 ml at a time.

Q162 A 50-year-old P3 presents complaining of urinary incontinence for the past two years. She leaks on coughing and sneezing, and has given up her aerobics classes. She empties her bladder frequently for fear of 'accidents'.

Q163 A 70-year-old P4 with an uterovaginal prolapse has a ring pessary fitted. She returns for follow up six weeks later and complains of frequency, dysuria, urgency and suprapubic discomfort.

Q164 A 29-year-old woman, who delivered vaginally seven days ago, attends her GP's surgery complaining of leakage of urine. She had a prolonged labour of 26 hours and was delivered by forceps under regional anaesthesia. She was discharged home 32 hours after delivery, having passed small amounts of urine on the post-natal ward.

Q165 A 30-year-old woman of African origin arrives in the UK as a refugee eight weeks after giving birth, and seeks medical help because of leakage of urine. She explains that she laboured over three days without medical assistance, and the baby was eventually stillborn. For the past four weeks she has been leaking urine continuously.

Theme: Abnormal vaginal bleeding

Options:

A   Dysfunctional uterine bleeding
B   Cervical carcinoma
C   Endometrial carcinoma
D   Uterine fibroids
E   Endometrial polyps
F   Trauma
G   Endometritis
H   Atrophic vaginitis
I   Foreign body
J   Anovulatory cycles

Lead-in:

For each of the following clinical presentations, please select the *most likely diagnosis* from the option list. Each option may be used once, more than once or not at all.

 A 16-year-old girl, whose menarche was one year ago, presents with heavy, irregular periods. Her cycles are 5–8/ 30–45, and she experiences passage of clots and flooding. She finds her periods embarrassing, but has not had to miss school so far. A recent Hb was 10.6 g/dl.

 A 71-year-old woman, who is 25 years post-menopausal, attends her GP's surgery for a 'flu jab'. She mentions finding some blood in her underwear occasionally. A transvaginal ultrasound is arranged by her GP, and reveals an endometrial thickness of 3.2 mm. Her Hb is 11.7 g/dl.

A 35-year-old woman attends her GP's surgery complaining of very heavy periods. She occasionally experiences soiling of her clothing and of the bed sheets. Her cycles are regular (4/29) with no intermenstrual or post-coital bleeding. On pelvic examination she has a normal-sized uterus and there is no evidence of adnexal pathology. Her Hb is 10.1 g/dl.

 A 30-year-old nulliparous woman of Afro-Caribbean origin complains of heavy vaginal bleeding. Her cycles are regular at 7/26, but extremely heavy, and she misses work during her periods. On examination her uterus is enlarged, irregular and non-tender. Her Hb is 8.9 g/dl.

 A 62-year-old obese woman with IDDM, who is 10 years post-menopausal, presents with heavy vaginal bleeding of 10 days' duration. A transvaginal ultrasound scan reveals an endometrial thickness of 17 mm.

Theme: Pelvic pain

Options:

A   MSU
B   Pregnancy test
C   CRP
D   FBC
E   Vaginal and endo-cervical swabs
F   Pelvic ultrasound scan
G   Renal tract ultrasound
H   CT of pelvis
I   Diagnostic laparoscopy
J   Culdocentesis

Lead-in:

For each of the clinical case scenarios below, select the *most useful investigation* from the list of options. Each option may be used once, more than once or not at all.

(Q171)   A 34-year-old nulliparous woman is seen in outpatients with a three-year history of painful periods. The pain starts three days before the onset of menstruation and lasts throughout. She has also developed deep dyspareunia. Pelvic examination reveals a fixed retroverted uterus.

(Q172)   A 19-year-old woman makes an appointment to see her GP. She is complaining of vague lower abdominal pain of two weeks' duration. There are no urinary symptoms, and her bowels are regular. She is on day 7 of her cycle, and she uses the combined oral contraceptive pill for contraception. She appears upset and confides that she has just found out that her boyfriend has been cheating on her. On examination her temperature is 37.4 °C and there is mild bilateral adnexal tenderness.

(Q173)   A 37-year-old woman was referred by her GP because of right iliac fossa pain. The pain started 24 hours ago. She is currently on the waiting list for IVF for tubal factor infertility. Her cycles occur every 28–45 days and she commonly gets intermenstrual bleeding. Her last menstrual period was 43 days ago. On examination her abdomen is soft with some tenderness in the right iliac fossa. Her uterus is of normal size and she has positive cervical excitation.

(Q174)   A 20-year-old nulliparous woman is referred by her GP with a two-week history of left iliac fossa pain. Although her cycles are usually regular she has now been amenorrhoeic for 10 weeks, and a serum b-HCG requested by her GP yesterday was <5 iU/l. On examination she is overweight, normotensive and not tachycardic; her abdomen is soft and there is marked left iliac fossa tenderness. Pelvic examination is difficult owing to the patient's habitus.

You are asked to review a 31-year-old nulliparous woman in the early pregnancy clinic. She first attended the clinic seven days ago at five weeks' amenorrhoea with mild right iliac fossa pain and spotting per vaginam. A transvaginal ultrasound scan has revealed an empty uterus, and three serum b-HCG levels performed at 48-hour intervals have been reported as 505, 700 and 895 iU/l, respectively.

12

Cancer in gynaecology

Theme: Treatment of female genital tract cancer

Options:

A   Radical hysterectomy
B   Wide local excision
C   Trachylectomy
D   Total abdominal hysterectomy and bilateral salpingo-oophorectomy
E   Radical vulvectomy
F   Ovarian cystectomy
G   Chemotherapy
H   Laparoscopically assisted vaginal hysterectomy
I   Vaginal hysterectomy
J   Radiotherapy

Lead-in:

For each of the clinical case scenarios below, select the *most appropriate treatment* from the list of options. Each option may be used once, more than once or not at all.

Q176 A 35-year-old multiparous woman undergoes cervical screening. As a result of an abnormal smear result and a subsequent biopsy of the transformation zone, squamous cell carcinoma of the cervix is diagnosed. Following clinical staging, she is found to have stage IIa cervical carcinoma.

Q177 A 35-year-old nulliparous woman undergoes cervical screening. As a result of an abnormal appearance of the cervix and a subsequent cervical biopsy, squamous cell carcinoma of the cervix is diagnosed. Following clinical staging, the tumour is found to extend bilaterally into the parametria, reaching the pelvic sidewalls.

Q178 A 55-year-old post-menopausal woman presents with a large abdominal mass. Ovarian carcinoma is suspected. She undergoes a laparotomy, where stage IV ovarian cancer is diagnosed.

Q179 A 65-year-old nulliparous woman, who is otherwise fit and well, presents with post-menopausal bleeding. Endometrial histology reveals well-differentiated adenocarcinoma.

Q180 A 73-year-old woman presents with vulval irritation and a 4×5 cm vulval lesion is found on inspection. There is also inguinal lymphadenopathy. A biopsy reveals squamous cell carcinoma of the vulva.

13

Screening and prevention

Theme: Women's health

Options:

A   Cancer of the colon
B   Endometrial carcinoma
C   Squamous cell carcinoma of the cervix
D   Germ cell ovarian tumour
E   Adenocarcinoma of the cervix
F   Breast cancer
G   Malignant melanoma
H   Choriocarcinoma
I   Epithelial ovarian tumour
J   Uterine sarcoma

Lead-in:

For each of the following cases, please select the *disease for which the patient is at particularly high risk* from the option list. Each option may be used once, more than once or not at all.

(Q181) A 33-year-old P1, who has had multiple sexual partners, and has used the combined oral contraceptive pill as the sole method of contraception for the past 18 years. Her BMI is 22 and she smokes 20 cigarettes per day.

(Q182) A 35-year-old woman suffers a spontaneous miscarriage at 13 weeks' gestation. Histology of products of conception reveals a complete mole.

(Q183) A 65-year-old nulliparous woman who has been on vaginal oestrogen cream for the past year for urogenital atrophy.

(Q184) A 58-year-old non-smoker with a BMI of 30, who has been on cyclical combined HRT for 12 years.

(Q185) A 35-year-old nulliparous women with a long history of primary infertility, who has undergone repeated cycles of ovarian stimulation.

Theme: Cervical screening

Options:

A   Repeat smear in three years
B   Repeat smear immediately
C   Refer for colposcopy
D   Repeat smear in six months
E   Discharge from screening programme
F   Radical hysterectomy
G   Repeat smear in one year
H   Repeat smear after antibiotic treatment
I   Repeat smear in two years
J   Refer for examination under anaesthesia

Lead-in:

For each of the following cases, please select the *most appropriate management* from the option list. Each option may be used once, more than once or not at all.

(Q186) A 35-year-old para 1, who has had multiple sexual partners, and had used the combined oral contraceptive pill as the sole method of contraception for the past 18 years. She had colposcopy following an abnormal smear 10 years ago, but her smears have been normal since. Three months ago she had a total abdominal hysterectomy for heavy periods.

(Q187) A 69-year-old nulliparous woman, whose menopause was 14 years ago, telephones her GP's surgery to enquire about the next appointment for a cervical smear. She has complied with the cervical screening programme in the past, and all her past smears have been reported as normal.

(Q188) A 27-year-old nullipara had a smear six weeks ago. She is a non-smoker, and has used barrier contraception for the past two years, having used the mini-pill previously. Her cervical smear report suggests 'moderate dyskaryosis'.

(Q189) A 49-year-old nulliparous woman, whose last menstrual period was 12 months ago, had a cervical smear taken two weeks ago. The smear report reads: 'No evidence of transformation zone sampling, inadequate smear'.

(Q190) A 30-year-old multipara attends the GP's surgery for a cervical smear. She had two smears, 12 and six months ago, which were reported as 'borderline'. The test is repeated, and the result is again 'borderline changes'.

14

Operative gynaecology

Theme: Peri-operative complications

Options:

A   Pulmonary embolus
B   Peritonitis
C   Uterine perforation
D   Aortic laceration
E   Gas embolus
F   Paralytic ileus
G   Bowel injury
H   Intestinal obstruction
I   Atelectasis
J   Urinary tract infection

Lead-in:

For each of the following cases, please select the *most likely underlying cause* from the option list. Each option may be used once, more than once or not at all.

 A 33-year-old parous woman with a BMI of 26 undergoes a laparotomy for stage II ovarian cancer. On the second post-operative day she complains of increased nausea and vomiting. Her abdomen appears distended, and there are no audible bowel sounds.

Q192 A 60-year-old nulliparous woman with a BMI of 36 undergoes an abdominal hysterectomy and bilateral salpingo-oophorectomy because of recurrent post-menopausal bleeding and endometrial hyperplasia. Her post-operative pain control is sub-optimal. On the second post-operative day she develops breathlessness, a tachypnoea of 24 bpm and mild pyrexia of 37.6 °C. Her blood pressure and pulse are normal, and on auscultation there is reduced air entry over both lung bases.

Q193 A 48-year-old parous woman with a BMI of 36 undergoes a vaginal hysterectomy and pelvic floor repair for prolapse. She makes good progress post-operatively and is discharged home on the fifth post-operative day, but before leaving the ward she complains of breathlessness. She appears tachypnoeic, her pulse is 120 bpm and her temperature is 37.4 °C. On auscultation her chest is clear, with normal air entry bilaterally.

Q194 A 30-year-old nulliparous woman with a BMI of 22 undergoes suction evacuation of the uterus because of a missed miscarriage at 12 weeks' gestation. During the procedure the cervix is noted to be difficult to dilate, and no tissue is obtained despite repeated attempts with the suction curette.

Q195 A 29-year-old woman with a BMI of 31 is undergoing a laparoscopy and dye pertubation because of primary infertility. Following the insertion of the sub-umbilical port the anaesthetist becomes concerned because of a rapid drop in the patient's blood pressure, initially with normal O_2 saturation. Her pulse rate increases from 60 bpm to 140 bpm within a five-minute period, and, although the surgeon discontinues CO_2 insufflation, her abdomen becomes increasingly distended and the patient appears shocked.

Theme: Surgical management in gynaecology

Options:

A Sub-total abdominal hysterectomy
B Vaginal hysterectomy
C Anterior colpoperineorrhaphy
D Colposuspension
E Total abdominal hysterectomy and bilateral oophorectomy
F Posterior colpoperineorrhaphy
G Laparoscopic salpingectomy
H Ovarian cystectomy
I Laparotomy and unilateral salpingectomy
J Hysterotomy

Lead-in:

For each of the following cases, please select the *most appropriate surgical management* from the option list. Each option may be used once, more than once or not at all.

 A 22-year-old woman is admitted to the A&E department with a two-hour history of severe abdominal pain. Although her menstrual cycles are usually regular at 4/29, her period is 10 days late. She has had vague abdominal discomfort and some spotting per vaginam for the past three days, but today the pain increased in severity. On examination her BP is 82/46 mmHg, her pulse is 120 bpm and her abdomen is tender with guarding and rebound tenderness. Her pregnancy test is faintly positive.

A 30-year-old woman presents with a six-month history of left iliac fossa pain. An ultra-sound scan reveals a left-sided simple ovarian cyst of 6 cm diameter. The right ovary appears normal and there is no free fluid in the pelvis. Her CA 125 level is 11 kU/l (5–35).

 A 60-year-old parous woman presents with lower abdominal discomfort. On ultrasound scan, there are bilateral, complex ovarian masses with thick, smooth capsules. There is no free fluid in the pelvis. The CA 125 level is 6 kU/l (5–35).

 A 30-year-old nulliparous woman is admitted to the gynaecology ward with left iliac fossa pain and spotting per vaginam. Her pregnancy test is faintly positive, although she cannot remember missing a period. Her BP is 124/66 mmHg and her pulse is 88 bpm. There is marked abdominal tenderness, but no guarding or rebound tenderness. On ultrasound scan there is no evidence of an intrauterine pregnancy, but there is what appears to be a gestational sac in the left adnexa with a fetal pole of about six weeks' gestation and fetal heart pulsations are seen.

 A 30-year-old woman, who is a Jehovah's Witness, requests surgical management of menorrhagia. Her periods are heavy, with the passage of large clots and flooding. Her haemoglobin is difficult to maintain with iron therapy. She has large fibroids, and multiple attempts at controlling her periods with conservative means, including medication, endometrial ablation and fibroid embolisation, have failed.

Theme: Devices and instruments in gynaecology

Options:

A

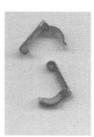

B

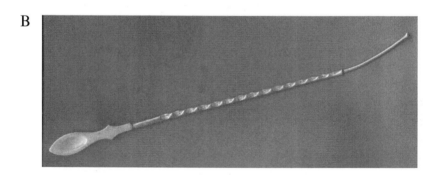

C

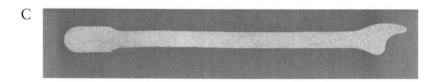

D

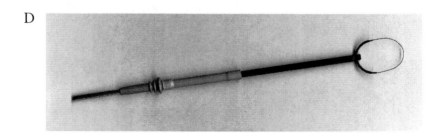

E

F

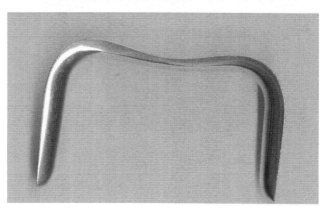

G

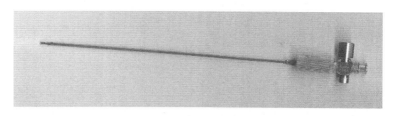

H

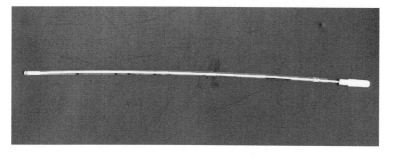

I

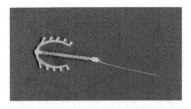

J

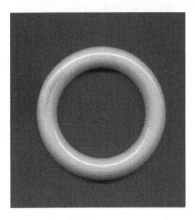

Lead-in:

For each of the following cases, please select the *most appropriate device or instrument* from the option list. Each option may be used once, more than once or not at all.

 A 30-year-old G4 P4 wishes to be sterilised. She is requesting information on the method of tubal occlusion.

 A 59-year-old woman who is 10 years post-menopausal and not on any hormone replacement therapy is attending her GP's surgery for a cervical smear.

 A 73-year-old woman with a second-degree utero-vaginal prolapse is requesting conservative management to avoid the risks of surgery.

A 66-year-old G5 P5 presents to a gynaecology clinic complaining of 'something coming down'. On inspection there is no obvious uterine prolapse, but you wish to establish whether or not there is a cystocoele.

 A 32-year-old parous woman has opted for a levonorgestrel intrauterine system to treat her heavy, regular periods. You are in the process of inserting the device, and wish to measure the length of the uterine cavity.

15

Therapeutics in gynaecology

Theme: Drug therapy in gynaecology

Options:

A   Metronidazole
B   GnRH agonist
C   Tranexamic acid
D   Dianette
E   Danazol
F   Doxycycline
G   Fluoxetine
H   Tolterodine
I   Bromocriptine
J   Metformin

Lead-in:

For each of the following patients, please select the *most appropriate therapeutic agent* from the option list. Each option may be used once, more than once or not at all.

A 30-year-old woman attends the GUM clinic because of an irritant vaginal discharge. *Trichomonas vaginalis* is diagnosed from a high vaginal swab.

 A 44-year-old nulliparous woman presents with urinary symptoms compatible with detrusor overactivity, which is confirmed on subsequent urodynamic testing.

 A 27-year-old nulliparous woman is referred to a gynaecology clinic with oligomenorrhoea and weight gain. She wishes to start a family, and has been trying to conceive for three years without success. An ultrasound scan of her pelvis reveals a pearl-string appearance of her ovaries.

 A 28-year-old woman is referred to a gynaecology clinic with oligomenorrhoea, weight gain and hirsutism. She uses condoms for contraception. Her sex hormone binding globulin levels are found to be low.

 A 39-year-old woman presents with secondary amenorrhoea. Investigations reveal raised prolactin levels and a pituitary microadenoma. Surgery is currently not indicated.

16

Ethics in obstetrics and gynaecology

Theme: Medico-legal and ethical principles 1

Options:

A   Confidentiality
B   Fraser (Gillick) competence
C   Non-maleficence
D   Negligence
E   Paternalism
F   Fidelity
G   Veracity
H   Battery
I   Beneficence
J   Bolam test

Lead-in:

For each of the following scenarios, please select the *most applicable principle* from the option list. Each option can be used once, more than once or not at all.

A 14-year-old girl attends a family planning clinic requesting emergency contraception. She discloses to the doctor that she has been sexually active with her 15-year-old boyfriend for the past three months.

 A 29-year-old primigravida goes into spontaneous labour at 39 weeks' gestation. She makes fast progress in labour, and active pushing is commenced two hours after admission; however, a fetal bradycardia occurs. A doctor is called, who decides to perform an instrumental delivery. The patient is distressed and in pain, and communication is difficult. She screams at the doctor to leave her alone and that she does not want to have an instrumental delivery. However, as the fetal heart is not recovering, the doctor feels it is essential to perform an instrumental delivery to save the baby's life, and performs a forceps delivery aided by staff with consent from the patient's husband.

 A 30-year-old G3 P2, who has had two previous un-complicated vaginal deliveries, goes into labour at 38 weeks' gestation. Her labour is prolonged, and the midwife is concerned about the fetal heart rate pattern. She repeatedly asks for the registrar to attend, but medical staff do not attend until an hour later. The baby is delivered by Caesarean section in very poor condition, and subsequently goes on to develop cerebral palsy.

 A 31-year-old nulliparous woman is diagnosed with stage IIa cervical cancer. The treatment options include a Wertheim hysterectomy or radiotherapy; you decide to schedule the patient for a Wertheim hysterectomy and inform the patient of your decision.

 A 26-year-old woman is admitted with acute PID and has to undergo a laparotomy and drainage of a pelvic abscess. She cancels her holiday because of her illness. A month later you receive a request from her insurance company to write a report detailing her medical problems that led to the cancellation.

Theme: Medico-legal and ethical principles 2

Options:

A   Confidentiality
B   Competence
C   Non-maleficence
D   Negligence
E   Paternalism
F   Autonomy
G   Veracity
H   Battery
I   Beneficence
J   Bolam test

Lead-in:

For each of the following scenarios, please select the *most relevant principle* from the option list. Each option can be used once, more than once or not at all.

 A 70-year-old woman is admitted to hospital for a laparotomy because of a pelvic mass, presumed to be ovarian in origin. Her family ask to speak to you, and request that you do not disclose the diagnosis to the patient if the tumour is malignant, because of their concerns for her psychological well-being.

 A 70-year-old woman is admitted to hospital for a laparotomy because of a pelvic mass, presumed to be ovarian in origin. Her family ask to speak to you and request that you disclose the diagnosis to them first.

A 30-year-old G1 P0 has a placenta praevia. She is scheduled to undergo an elective Caesarean section at 39 weeks. She informs you that she is a Jehovah's Witness and that she will not accept a blood transfusion under any circumstances. During the Caesarean section she develops a massive haemorrhage, and despite prompt and decisive management, she dies.

 A 21-year-old woman, who is educationally subnormal, is brought in by ambulance with abdominal pain at 36 weeks' gestation. She appears to be in early labour, but the baby is presenting by the breech. Her legal guardian, who usually attends all hospital visits with her, is delayed. You feel that she requires a Caesarean section immediately and talk to her about the need for surgery and about signing a consent form herself.

 A 26-year-old woman is admitted to A&E with what appears to be a ruptured ectopic pregnancy. She is hypovolaemic and she has lost consciousness; communication to obtain consent is impossible. You decide to proceed to an immediate laparotomy to save her life.

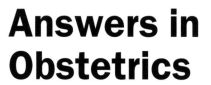

Answers in Obstetrics

17

Normal pregnancy

Theme: Physiological changes in pregnancy

 I

This is a healthy woman in the second trimester of pregnancy. Her low blood pressure is the result of peripheral vascular dilation. Whilst the rise in cardiac output compensates to a degree for the drop in vascular resistance, the net effect is usually a reduction in blood pressure, with a nadir in the second trimester. BP tends to increase again in the third trimester.

 F

This is normocytic, normochromic anaemia. In the context of a normal pregnancy, the underlying cause in the third trimester is most likely to be the increased circulating volume. There is an increase in red cell mass in pregnancy, but the net effect tends to be that of haemodilution by the relatively greater increase in plasma volume.

 B

Glycosuria in pregnancy can be physiological as the renal threshold for glucose is reduced. However, recurrent glycosuria in the late-second and third trimesters needs to be investigated to exclude gestational diabetes. Any glycosuria in the first and early-second trimesters must be investigated, as it may be a sign of pre-existing, as yet undiagnosed, diabetes mellitus.

G

Because of delayed gastric emptying during labour (and in pregnancy), these women received intrapartum H2 inhibitors to decrease gastric acid secretion. Where the need for general anaesthesia arises, pregnant women have a higher risk of failed intubation and aspiration of gastric contents than the non-pregnant population, and mortality from Mendelssohn syndrome is high. Other prophylactic measures include fasting in labour, administration of sodium citrate, application of cricoid pressure at intubation and use of cuffed endotracheal tubes, and the use of regional rather than general anaesthesia where possible.

 J

The combination of smooth muscle relaxation and the mass effect of the pregnant uterus in late pregnancy can lead to venous stasis and the formation of varicosities in dependent areas. Varicose veins are not uncommon in pregnancy.

Theme: Pregnancy milestones

 D

First maternal perception of fetal movements, also termed 'quickening', occurs around 14–16 weeks in parous women and at 18–20 weeks in first-time mothers.

 G

The description is that of mood symptoms which can accompany the 'baby blues', commonly occurring in more than 50% of women. Peak onset is between days 2–4 post-partum, and symptoms usually last up to a week. Other symptoms include emotional lability, sadness, insomnia, difficulty concentrating and headaches. Treatment is supportive. Mood disturbances also accompany the much more serious post-natal depression, where symptoms are sustained, with a peak incidence at 3–4 weeks post-partum.

I

The fundus is palpable at the xiphisternum at approximately 38 weeks' gestation, and it 'drops' thereafter with the engagement of the presenting part.

 I

In nulliparous women the presenting part should engage by 36–38 weeks; if engagement does not occur, placenta praevia needs to be excluded. Less common causes of non-engagement include large cervical fibroids and, rarely, fetal abnormality such as hydrocephalus. In multiparous women the presenting part may remain high until the onset of labour.

 A

The uterine fundus is usually palpable at the level of the umbilicus at approximately 22 weeks' gestation.

18

Ante-natal care and pre-natal diagnosis

Theme: Ante-natal screening and diagnosis

 C

This patient wants to know whether or not her baby is affected, which means you need to offer her a diagnostic rather than a screening test. She wishes to have a test as soon as possible; a chorionic villous sample (CVS) can be taken after 10 weeks' gestation, whereas an amniocentesis is offered from 15 weeks onwards. An earlier CVS carries a risk of limb reduction defects, whereas an amniocentesis performed before 15 weeks has a higher risk of miscarriage.

 E

Women with IDDM who have poor periconceptual control have a higher risk of fetal abnormality, in particular congenital heart defects. Fetal cardiac echo is therefore the most useful test in this scenario. A nuchal translucency (NT) test would also be useful; however, this patient is already 22 weeks pregnant and NT is performed at 11–13 weeks' gestation.

B

This patient wishes to have some information about her risk of carrying a Down's syndrome baby, which means she can be offered a screening test. At that gestation NT would be the best option.

 J

A uterine artery Doppler would provide useful information in this case. High resistance flow in the uterine artery and so-called 'notching' in the waveform results from inadequate conversion of the spiral arteries to a high-capacity, low-resistance circulation. Uterine artery notching at 20–24 weeks' gestation is associated with an increased risk of IUGR and pre-eclampsia later in pregnancy in a high-risk population.

 A

This patient wishes to have a diagnosis rather than a risk assessment; at her gestational age she can be offered an amniocentesis.

Theme: Aneuploidy and genetic disorders

This question is fairly difficult for undergraduates, and would certainly come under 'further reading' rather than 'essential knowledge'. Questions of this type may be used to 'pick out' students who may be considered for a distinction. However, the information provided in most of the cases below (at least the Down's syndrome and molar pregnancy scenarios) should be familiar to the majority of students.

(A16) A

The patient in this case scenario is at increased risk of fetal aneuploidy based on her age. The described sonographic markers are most likely to occur with trisomy 18 (Edwards' syndrome). Choroid plexus cysts are seen in 25% of fetuses with T18. Other associated features may include neural tube defects (20%), exomphalos (25%), facial clefts, diaphragmatic hernias and cardiac malformations. Differential diagnosis must include trisomy 13 (Patau syndrome), where brain malformations are more common (holoprosencephaly in 40%) as are central facial clefts (45%).

(A17) B

Generalised fetal oedema and cystic hygroma (cystic swelling at the back of the fetal neck), although not diagnostic, are typical of monosomy X0 (Turner's syndrome). In the newborn period, dorsal pedal oedema is often observed. Other features apparent after birth and later in childhood/adolescence include a webbed neck, shield thorax, a wide carrying angle and short stature. Coarctation of the aorta and other malformations of the left heart, such as aortic valve stenosis, can occur.

(A18) H

Nuchal translucency screening detects approximately 80% of aneuploidies (mainly trisomy 21); increased nuchal translucency can also be associated with cardiac malformations. In this case, the soft markers detected during the second trimester detailed ultrasound suggest the presence of T21 (Down's syndrome).

(A19) I

The clue in this case scenario is in the early-onset pre-eclampsia, which would not normally be expected to occur before 24 weeks' gestation. It can occur early in the presence of a molar pregnancy. Triploidy, where an entire extra set of chromosomes results in 69 chromosomes instead of the usual 46, can result in molar changes in the placenta as well as an abnormal fetus, and pre-eclampsia or a thyrotoxic-like state can ensue.

C

Achondroplasia is the most common autosomal dominant form of non-lethal dwarfism, and it occurs in 1:1000 to 1:2000 live births. The clue in the case scenario is given by the average measurements of head and abdomen compared to the disproportionately short limbs. Other ultrasonographic features may include a prominent forehead (frontal bossing) and a small chest. Down's syndrome can be associated with a short femur, but a significant shortening of other long bones, in particular in the upper limbs, would not be expected.

Theme: Ante-natal risk assessment

 H

Multiple previous Caesarean sections increase the risk of a placenta praevia. Additionally, where the placenta implants on the anterior uterine wall over the thinner myometrium of the scar region, it can become morbidly adherent and, in fact, breach the serosal surface of the uterus. This is a serious, potentially life-threatening situation which can result in massive obstetric haemorrhage. A hysterectomy is often required to prevent maternal death.

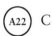 C

This patient appears to have developed recurrent glycosuria in the early third trimester, as it was detected during three consecutive ante-natal visits. This may reflect impaired glucose tolerance (gestational diabetes). As glucose crosses the placenta, fetal hyper-glycaemia and hyperinsulinism with consequent macrosomia can ensue. Fetal macrosomia is seen as the primary consequence of gestational diabetes. There is controversy about other indices of fetal and neonatal morbidity and mortality, and macrosomia is therefore the best answer in this question.

D

This woman reports watery vaginal discharge since her amniocentesis at 20 weeks' gestation. This implies a continued amniotic fluid leak for the past seven weeks, resulting in oligohydramnios. The lack of liquor at such early gestation will affect fetal lung development, resulting in pulmonary hypoplasia. Other possible consequences of severe oligohydramnios for the developing fetus include postural limb defects and Potter facies.

 G

The most obvious risk to this pregnancy relates to maternal use of high-dose anticonvulsants, therefore 'neural tube defect' is the best answer from the option list.

 B

The most likely diagnosis is obstetric cholestasis (OC), although other causes of pruritus in pregnancy would have to be excluded. Given the working diagnosis, stillbirth or intrauterine fetal death will be the most likely risk from the option list. Other risks of OC include fetal distress, meconium-stained liquor, prematurity (often iatrogenic) and post-partum haemorrhage owing to reduced levels of vitamin K-dependent coagulation factors.

Theme: Teratogens

 B

Patients with prosthetic valves require full anticoagulation. Outside pregnancy, the anticoagulant of choice is warfarin. Warfarin is contraindicated in the first and third trimesters, but can be prescribed in the second trimester and to breast-feeding mothers. In the first trimester its teratogenic effects include abnormalities of cartilage and bone; in the third trimester the adverse effects relate to the fact that warfarin crosses the placenta and anticoagulates the fetus, potentially causing intracranial haemorrhage.

E

The most likely drug to produce the described maternal and fetal effects is phenytoin. Phenytoin can lead to gingival hyperplasia in its users. The constellation of facial clefting and congenital heart defects suggests a possible anticonvulsant syndrome. Lamotrigine, the other anticonvulsant on the list, is not known to be associated with gingival hyperplasia, and, so far, it appears to have a favourable teratogenic profile. As this patient has not sought ante-natal care, she would not have received advice on the type and dosage of her anti-epileptic drugs.

 J

Fetal growth restriction, microcephaly, mid-face hypoplasia and mental retardation are features of the fetal alcohol syndrome. The supporting facts in the scenario are the stigmata of liver disease in the mother.

 H

The patient in this case scenario has a history of chlamydial infection. The antibiotics of choice outside pregnancy are tetracyclines, such as doxycycline. There is a theoretical risk of discolouration and dysplasia of teeth and bones in the fetus. Whilst tetracyclines would not normally be prescribed in pregnancy, the mother may have become exposed if pregnancy was not excluded prior to the treatment.

 D

Although rubella immunisation is widespread, a small proportion of women of childbearing age fail to acquire immunity. Congenital rubella can result in deafness, blindness and mental retardation, particularly where exposure occurred in the first trimester. Cytomegalovirus is a close contender for the right answer; however, most babies with congenital CMV are asymptomatic at birth. Those with symptoms usually present with petechial haemorrhages, DIC, hepatic impairment or failure and bacterial superinfection. They can also subsequently demonstrate sensorineural deafness, but cardiac malformations are not a feature of congenital CMV.

19

Common presentations in pregnancy

Theme: Early pregnancy

 J

Resolution of pregnancy symptoms, together with a smaller-than-expected uterine size, is suspicious of a failed intrauterine pregnancy. In the absence of vaginal bleeding, the most likely diagnosis is a missed miscarriage, which can be entirely asymptomatic.

 I

Excessive vomiting in pregnancy and a large-for-gestational-age uterus can indicate a multiple pregnancy or a hydatidiform mole. Both conditions are associated with high levels of human chorionic gonadotrophin, resulting in increased nausea and vomiting, and the uterine size is larger than expected.

 A

Painless vaginal bleeding in pregnancy is usually considered to be a symptom of a threatened miscarriage. In this case scenario, the presence of the fetal heart on auscultation is reassuring, and confirms an ongoing pregnancy.

F

Vaginal bleeding and lower abdominal pain, in particular with passage of clots, suggest that the pregnancy may no longer be viable. The fact that the bleeding has settled spontaneously after the expulsion of large clots at the given gestation makes the diagnosis of complete miscarriage very likely. This is supported by the finding of a normal-sized uterus – this should be taken to mean a uterus that is not enlarged – and a closed cervical os.

 C

The patient is this scenario has suffered a first-trimester pregnancy loss in the form of an anembryonic gestation. She had medical intervention to expedite uterine evacuation, in this case a medical evacuation. Her symptoms have become progressively worse since the intervention, suggesting the presence of retained products of conception. Incomplete miscarriage, on the other hand, is a term used to describe an ongoing miscarriage independent of any medical intervention.

Theme: Abdominal pain 1

 I

Torsion of an ovarian cyst is the most likely diagnosis amongst the options given. The pain is intermittent, confined to the LIF, and there are signs of peritoneal irritation. Pain from a UTI or pyelonephritis is unlikely to cause peritoneal irritation; red degeneration of a fibroid is likely to result in constant pain. Pre-term labour can cause intermittent pain; however, there would not be peritonism and the pain is unlikely to be unilateral.

 C

The patient is this case scenario is from an ethnic background with a higher risk of fibroids, and, furthermore, her uterus is measured large for dates and is described as irregular in outline. This points to red degeneration of a fibroid as the most likely underlying cause for the patient's pain.

A38 D

The clue is this case scenario lies in the absence of any positive findings and the fact that the patient is engaging in strenuous physical activity. However, remember that musculoskeletal pain has to be a diagnosis of exclusion.

 A39 E

The patient is this scenario is most likely to have appendicitis. Remember that the appendix is displaced upwards by the enlarged uterus. Other clues include age, duration and type of symptoms, and pyrexia. Pyelonephritis would be a differential diagnosis; however, peritonism would again be less likely.

 A40 H

The abdominal pain here is recurring in regular intervals, it is associated with backache and the presenting part has engaged despite the early gestation. Urinalysis reveals + of proteinuria, which is often contamination from increased vaginal discharge/ show in labour. There are no nitrites or leucocytes in the sample, making a UTI less likely, although a UTI can trigger uterine contractions.

Theme: Abdominal pain 2

 A41 E

The patient is this scenario is most likely to have a torting ovarian cyst (see answer 36 above). The most useful investigation in this case would be a pelvic ultrasound.

 A42 E

Uterine fibroids are best diagnosed by ultrasound of the uterus (see answer 37).

A43 H

The patient has upper abdominal pain, vomiting and there is right upper quadrant tenderness. Cholecystitis may occur in pregnancy and the patient should therefore be investigated appropriately. The most useful test from the list will be liver function tests; the patient will also require an upper abdominal ultrasound.

A44 A

The case scenario leads us to the diagnosis of appendicitis. As there is peritonism, an FBC will be useful; although white cell count can be raised in pregnancy, we would expect it to be disproportionately raised here. The utility of pelvic ultrasound to diagnose appendicitis at 26 weeks' gestation is debatable; the diagnosis will have to be made on clinical grounds.

A45 B

The presence of uterine tightenings and irritability is commonly seen in association with maternal infection. In pregnancy, UTIs are common and can result in uterine activity. This is supported by the urinalysis result, and a culture of a mid-stream specimen of urine would be the most useful investigation. There is no added benefit from performing an ultrasound scan in this situation; in the absence of pyrexia or ruptured membranes FBC is of limited value.

Theme: Anaemia

 E

The patient is this case scenario has a history of alcohol abuse. Under these circumstances folate deficiency is common, resulting in a macrocytic rather than microcytic anaemia.

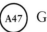 **G**

The patient in this case scenario has severe pre-eclampsia and symptoms suggestive of HELLP (haemolysis, elevated liver enzymes, low platelets) syndrome, such as RUQ tenderness and vomiting. The haemolysis would affect the FBC in terms of reduction in Hb and haematocrit, and there would be a marked reduction in platelets. In option F the platelets are mildly reduced, but Hb and haematocrit are normal, which is not compatible with significant haemolysis.

 B

This patient is likely to have a b-thalassaemia trait. This can be associated with a mild to moderate anaemia with disproportionately low MCV and MCH.

 D

The patient with hyperemesis is likely to be substantially dehydrated, resulting in haemoconcentration, as evidenced by a high Hb and haematocrit. There is not likely to be an infectious cause here, and WCC and platelets would be expected to be in the normal range for pregnancy.

 J

This woman has puerperal sepsis. She is likely to be dehydrated and have features of a response to infection, such as raised WCC and thrombocytosis. Whilst one would expect signs of haemoconcentration in the early post-partum period, and her Hb and haematocrit may not be substantially raised even with a degree of dehydration, often there is anaemia relating to recent pregnancy and blood loss during confinement, which means Hb and haematocrit may be low in the puerperium.

Theme: Shortness of breath

 C

This case scenario is set out to guide you to the diagnosis of venous thrombo-embolism (VTE). The patient has a number of demographic and situational risk factors (age, high BMI, high parity, smoking, pregnancy, period of restricted mobility). Under these circumstances, pulmonary embolism has to be the leading differential diagnosis until proven otherwise. You are further helped here by the clinical findings of tachypnoea, mild tachycardia and decreased O_2 saturations in room air. Remember that VTE is the leading cause of maternal mortality in the UK, and has to be considered in cases much less obvious than the one above!

 J

This patient clearly has an asthma attack. First presentation during pregnancy is not unusual, particularly in a younger patient. Apart from the clinical presentation, a further clue is given by the atopic history. Most medications used to treat asthma are suitable for use in pregnancy, including inhaled and/or oral steroids where indicated. A common reason for deterioration of asthma in pregnancy is poor maternal compliance with, or discontinuation of, drugs – often on medical advice – because of concerns about harmful effects on the fetus. It is essential that good asthma control be maintained throughout pregnancy.

 G

This patient is presenting with typical symptoms of anaemia in the third trimester of pregnancy. Although 'dilutional' anaemia is physiological in pregnancy, it is rarely severe enough to cause significant symptoms; however, iron deficiency anaemia commonly co-exists and of course other causes of anaemia must be borne in mind. The red cell indices should help in the differential diagnostic process as in non-pregnant individuals, and further investigations should be performed as indicated.

B

The most likely diagnosis in this case is chest infection. The patient's background makes her more likely to seek treatment for respiratory tract infections and perhaps have a degree of suppressed immunity if blood-borne diseases co-exist. The clinical signs suggest right basal pneumonia. Appropriate investigations, including a chest X-ray, have to be performed to confirm the diagnosis; the patient should be offered screening for blood-borne diseases if not already done in early pregnancy.

 D

The most likely diagnosis is hyperventilation; this is supported by the lack of clinical signs, and the history leading up to the onset of symptoms and of tingling in the patient's hands. Perioral numbness would be another symptom to ask about. Bear in mind that hyperventilation may co-exist with other pathology such as pulmonary embolism, and careful assessment is required in all cases.

Theme: Reduced fetal movements

 B

There is likely to be substantial maternal anxiety here. The obstetric descriptors suggest that this woman may have suffered a number of pregnancy losses. The fact that she presents at this early gestation, and after only a four-hour interval, suggests that anxiety will be heightened.

 A

The clues to the cause of reduced maternal perception of fetal movements in this case are the large-for-dates uterus and the presence of glycosuria. This suggests that the patient has undiagnosed gestational diabetes with polyhydramnios, which may result in reduced perception of fetal movements by the mother. For those of you who have done further reading, option C (fetal dyskinesia)

may appear plausible also. Fetal dyskinesia syndromes (FDS) are a group of disorders which may affect fetal motility for a variety of musculoskeletal or neurological problems, such as severe arthrogryposis, for example. Where fetal swallowing is impaired in FDS polyhydramnios may also develop; however, the glycosuria in this case points to hyperglycaemia as an underlying cause.

 E

The fetus in this case scenario is clearly compromised as evidenced by a non-reassuring CTG. The most likely reason for this is severe intrauterine growth restriction associated with maternal preeclampsia.

 F

The reason for reduced fetal movements in this case is evident from the presence of pain, and the findings of a tense and tender uterus with maternal hypotension and tachycardia. The patient appears to have a concealed placental abruption. Whilst one would anticipate severe pain in association with an abruption, the symptoms can be more insidious, particularly with a posteriorly located placenta. There is also evidence of fetal compromise in this case, namely fetal bradycardia.

 C

This is an example of fetal dyskinesia disorders affecting the ability of the fetus to move. One would anticipate abnormal posture or limb position, abnormal movement patterns and possibly polyhydramnios on ultrasound.

Theme: Vaginal bleeding

 A

This should be an easy diagnosis to make. Ante-partum haemorrhage associated with a tender, tense uterus and maternal haemodynamic compromise is likely to be the result of placental abruption. In this case the bleeding is revealed, making the diagnosis more obvious.

C

The mother in this case scenario is not compromised; however, there is fetal bradycardia. Onset of painless ante-partum haemorrhage immediately following rupture of membranes is suggestive of vasa praevia, where fetal blood vessels, usually coursing through the umbilical cord directly to the placenta, leave the protective confines of the cord too early and run through the fetal membranes to the placenta. If membrane rupture occurs at this site the vessels rupture and the fetus exsanguinates.

 E

Multiple previous Caesarean sections increase the risk of placenta praevia. Typically, there is painless ante-partum haemorrhage without fetal compromise, as the bleeding is of maternal origin. Fetal compromise can be present occasionally as a result of maternal haemodynamic decompensation, but is not a typical feature.

 I

Recurrent post-coital bleeding can be a sign of a cervical lesion. Women with HIV, particularly those originating from the developing world and thus not offered cervical screening, are at particularly high risk of cervical cancer.

 D

This patient gives a history of irritant vaginal discharge, suggesting the presence of vulvo-vaginitis. Where particularly severe, it can give rise to bloodstained vaginal discharge.

20

Complications of pregnancy

Theme: Hypertensive disorders

 I

This patient with pre-eclampsia appears to have been overloaded with fluid, resulting in pulmonary oedema. The diagnosis can be made on clinical grounds, but should be confirmed by a chest X-ray. Remember that the leading causes of death among pre-eclamptic women in the UK are intracranial haemorrhage (poor control of blood pressure) and pulmonary complications, where inadequate fluid management is often a contributory factor.

 C

This patient is normotensive and non-proteinuric, suggesting that the oedema may be physiological – this is supported by the site of the oedema. However, she has a symphysio-fundal height (SFH) outside the range for this gestation. The most useful investigation in this case will be an ultrasound scan to assess fetal growth. SFH measurements have relatively low sensitivity and specificity, and sonographic measurements are the gold standard for the diagnosis of fetal growth restriction.

J

This patient has symptoms of a urinary tract infection, and the urinalysis results support this. The midwife has cautiously referred her for a hospital assessment because of proteinuria; however, the most useful investigation will be a culture of a mid-stream specimen of urine.

 G

This patient's main risk in this pregnancy is recurrent severe early onset pre-eclampsia and IUGR. At 22 weeks' gestation, the most useful investigation will be a uterine artery Doppler, which has a good predictive value in high-risk women of early onset PET and IUGR. In the first and early-second trimesters the trophoblast invades the uterine vasculature (spiral arteries) and destroys the *muscularis media* layer, thus making the vessels 'floppy' and less able to constrict. This ensures that the pregnancy will have a high-capacity, low-resistance circulation to draw on later on. If these changes are absent or incomplete, the risk of PET and/or IUGR increases. The uterine artery Doppler waveform at 20–24 weeks' gestation is a reflection of whether these changes have occurred.

 B

The patient has been diagnosed as pre-eclamptic, suggesting that she has hypertension and proteinuria. The main issue in terms of regional anaesthesia here is the exclusion of thrombocytopenia, which can occasionally complicate pre-eclampsia; a low platelet count would increase the risk of epidural haematoma and, depending on severity, may be considered a contraindication to epidural analgesia.

Theme: Diabetes in pregnancy

 D

This patient has impaired glucose tolerance; during pregnancy this is treated as gestational diabetes. The first intervention under these circumstances would be dietary adjustment; insulin treatment would be considered if dietary control is sub-optimal.

G

The fact that this woman has pre-existing Type 1 diabetes implies that she is likely to be on insulin therapy already. There is marked macrosomia, and the best management strategy under these circumstances is to deliver the baby by Caesarean section, to avoid the significant risk of shoulder dystocia.

 A

The patient has overt diabetes, as indicated by the high fasting and two-hour blood sugar levels. Under these circumstances the patient is likely to require dietary modification *and* insulin treatment to minimise the effect of hyperglycaemia on the fetus.

 F

The main problem described in this case is threatened pre-term labour at 29 weeks' gestation, and the most appropriate step would be to administer ante-natal steroids to augment fetal lung maturation. The fact that there is gestational diabetes complicates the issue somewhat, because steroids are likely to increase maternal blood sugar levels. Regular maternal blood sugar monitoring should to be carried out for 48 hours following the administration of steroids to see if insulin treatment will be required. In patients with unstable diabetes an insulin sliding scale may be required; however, it will usually suffice to increase the usual insulin dosage by approximately 15% for 2–3 days.

 E

Reduced fetal movements near term are always to be taken seriously. However, in this patient they are of particular concern because she has already had a stillbirth, and maternal diabetes mellitus is associated with an increased risk of intrauterine death. As this woman is parous and the baby is of average size, induction of labour at the earliest opportunity would be the most appropriate management in this case.

Theme: Collapse

 F

The patient in this scenario collapsed whilst standing in a queue, having felt faint and dizzy. The most likely explanation is postural hypotension, which can occur in association with prolonged standing, or with fast 'standing up'. In a classical vaso-vagal episode a slower pulse rate should be anticipated because of the vagal effects on the heart.

 G

Collapse with cyanosis and significant hypotension is suggestive of an embolic event. The patient in the case scenario is bleeding from puncture sites, which indicates developing disseminated intravascular coagulation (DIC). This is typical in Amniotic Fluid Embolism (AFE), rather than thrombotic embolism. The patient's risk factors for AFE are polyhydramnios and precipitate labour. Uterine inversion can also cause sudden collapse with haemodynamic instability and post-partum haemorrhage; however, it is rarely cyanotic and DIC may develop in due course as a result of the haemorrhage rather than as an early feature.

 D

Intracranial haemorrhage, resulting from a hypertensive crisis, is the most likely cause of this patient's collapse. Eclampsia usually presents with tonic clonic seizures rather than sudden loss of consciousness.

 A

This patient suffered a tonic–clonic seizure. Although epilepsy is a differential diagnosis, in the presence of hypertension and proteinuria one has to assume this is eclampsia until proven otherwise.

J

Difficulty delivering the placenta and continuing attempts at controlled cord traction can result in uterine inversion. Typically, the patient becomes hypotensive and shocked, and often post-partum haemorrhage ensues. On palpation the uterine fundus is no longer identifiable abdominally, and on pelvic examination there is a vaginal mass with or without the placenta attached, consistent with a uterine inversion.

Theme: Obstetric haemorrhage

 G

In terms of differential diagnosis, the most useful investigation is going to be an ultrasound scan looking for placental location. This patient may have a placenta praevia. Multiple previous Caesarean sections increase the risk of placenta praevia; in addition, the bleeding here is painless and there is no fetal compromise. A CTG is likely to be performed here, but, in the presence of normal fetal movements and a normal fetal heart rate on auscultation, an ultrasound will be more informative.

 C

This patient, who smokes, has an ante-partum haemorrhage associated with pain. Placental abruption is therefore quite likely, and fetal compromise can ensue. The fact that fetal movements are reduced indicates that fetal well-being should be assessed as a matter of urgency. Maternal well-being always has to be assessed first; however, the case scenario implies that this has been done and that the mother is stable. Maternal observations have to be made at frequent intervals because collapse can occur rapidly and the usual precautions (IV access, intravenous fluid, access to blood products, etc.) should be taken in all cases of significant obstetric haemorrhage or suspected placental abruption.

(A83) E

As in the theme on vaginal bleeding earlier, the suspicion here is that a cervical malignancy may have arisen in this HIV-positive patient. A cervical smear is the investigation of choice; practically, the cervix would be inspected first and, if a macroscopic lesion is present, cervical biopsy may be more appropriate.

(A84) F

This patient, who has had an uneventful pregnancy, is near term and is experiencing uterine contractions. She must be asked about any fresh, frank bleeding; however, the passage of bloodstained mucus is compatible with a show and no investigations are necessary in this case. The patient would be advised to present to the hospital when contractions are regular.

(A85) A

Here, we have a rhesus-negative patient who has had recurrent vaginal bleeding and has repeatedly failed to present to the hospital or attend ante-natal clinic appointments. There is a possibility that she has developed anti-D antibodies, which can cross the placenta and cause haemolysis. The first step would be to check her antibody titre; an ultrasound would be helpful if there is an increase in the titre or if there are clinical signs of fetal anaemia. In the presence of Rh isoimmunisation, fetal hydrops and polyhydramnios may develop, in which case a large-for-dates symphysio-fundal height or reduced fetal movements may be described.

Theme: Fetal growth disorders

(A86) I

The constellation of symptoms in the newborn, including intrauterine growth restriction, petechiae, jaundice and hepatosplenomegaly are typical of congenital infection. The most common causative agent is cytomegalovirus.

H

The patient in this case scenario is homeless, with a low BMI – suggesting a degree of self-neglect. She has failed to attend antenatal care. The baby is growth-restricted and displays symptoms compatible with withdrawal. These circumstantial factors suggest a patient with a substance abuse problem. Vasoactive substances, such as cocaine or amphetamines, are more likely to lead to 'vascular' type complications such as IUGR, placental abruption and hypertension than are marijuana or heroin.

 J

The history of recurrent miscarriages and venous thromboembolism suggests an underlying prothrombotic condition, which can, in turn, affect placentation and result in IUGR and other obstetric complications such as placental abruption, pre-eclampsia or stillbirth. Antiphospholipid syndrome is an 'acquired' thrombophilia, in contrast to familial (genetic) thrombophilias such as protein C or S deficiency, antithrombin III deficiency and factor V Leiden mutation.

 C

A macrosomic baby with recurrent neonatal hypoglycaemia suggests undiagnosed maternal diabetes. Maternal risk factors in this case include age and a high BMI.

 G

The woman in the case scenario is of Indo-Asian origin and has a low BMI; both are factors that suggest the baby is likely to be constitutionally small rather than growth-restricted. Misclassification as IUGR can be avoided if customised birthweight centile charts are used, adjusted for ethnicity, maternal size, parity and fetal gender.

21
Therapeutics in pregnancy and puerperium

Theme: Drug therapy in pregnancy and puerperium

 F

Lamotrigine is currently the drug of choice in women of reproductive age, as it appears to have a more favourable teratogenic profile.

 B

This patient with pre-eclampsia presents with symptoms of fulminating disease, which can result in eclampsia. The 'Magpie' trial has shown that the risk of seizures can be reduced if intravenous magnesium sulphate is administered. Magnesium sulphate has also been shown to reduce the risk of recurrent seizures in eclampsia, and it is the first-line drug in the management of eclamptic seizures. It also has a positive effect on blood pressure: magnesium is a 'natural calcium antagonist' and thus produces a degree of vasodilation and blood pressure reduction. However, as the effect is small, magnesium sulphate is not used as an antihypertensive agent. Intravenous antihypertensives are usually required in this situation.

E

The likely diagnosis in this case is pulmonary embolism. Warfarin is contraindicated in the third trimester of pregnancy as it crosses the placenta and anticoagulates the fetus. Low molecular weight heparin is the most appropriate treatment.

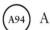 A

Hypertension in the first trimester of pregnancy suggests pre-existing hypertension, as gestational hypertension and pre-eclampsia rarely develop before 24 weeks of pregnancy. Provided hypertension is confirmed by repeated measurements, the drug of choice from the option list is methyldopa. Atenolol is not used in pregnancy as it can lead to fetal growth impairment, and ACE inhibitors may result in fetal renal failure and intrauterine fetal death. Other drugs which may be used under these circumstances include nifedipine and labetalol.

 C

Uterotonic drugs used for active management of the third stage of labour include oxytocin, ergometrin and a mixture of the two, syntometrin. Ergometrin is contraindicated in cardiac disease, as it can result in systemic hypertension. Oxytocin may be used, but with caution as it can have cardiac side effects also.

22

Labour, delivery and puerperium

Theme: Intrapartum assessment

 I

Against the background of the fast progress in labour, it is unlikely that there is a malpresentation (brow, face, breech or shoulder presentation) or malposition (occipito-posterior or occipito-transverse position). The most likely finding on vaginal examination will be that of a vertex presentation in an occipito-anterior position. In this position, the fetal occiput (identified by the posterior fontanelle and lambdoid stutures) can be palpated anteriorly under the maternal symphysis pubis.

 D

Pre-labour rupture of membranes and slow progress in a nullipara are typical in the presence of an occipito-posterior (OP) position. This is further supported by the continued severe backache the woman is experiencing throughout labour. Labour often has to be augmented under these circumstances, and effective analgesia, often in the form of a regional block, is required. A substantial proportion of OP positions will rotate into occipito-anterior position in due course, provided contractions are effective. The diagnosis of OP position is made by identifying the relevant landmarks of the fetal occiput (the posterior fontanelle and lambdoid sutures) oriented posteriorly in the maternal pelvis.

B

A markedly deflexed head results in a face presentation. Face presentation may be confused with a breech presentation occasionally, but can be identified by the chin (mentum), nasal bridge and orbital ridges. The fact that the patient delivered rapidly suggests that this was a mento-anterior face presentation, as a mento-posterior presentation is incompatible with vaginal delivery unless rotation occurs.

 A

The position described here is a right occipito-transverse position, which means that the fetal occiput is positioned on the maternal right.

 E

As discussed above, a markedly deflexed head suggests a face presentation. A high order multipara would be expected to deliver vaginally in the presence of a mento-anterior face presentation; therefore, the most likely position here is mento-posterior (fetal chin pointing to maternal sacrum). This is incompatible with vaginal delivery and obstructed labour can ensue. In the presence of a mento-posterior position the fetal head is maximally extended and the 'extension' step in the mechanism of labour cannot take place. In a mento-anterior position the fetal chin can get around the maternal symphysis pubis; the fetal head is, in fact, flexed in the 'extension' step, and vaginal delivery is possible.

Theme: Management of labour

 A

A transverse lie in established labour poses a risk to the mother (obstructed labour, ruptured uterus) and to the fetus (cord prolapse). A delivery by Caesarean section is therefore indicated under these circumstances.

J

This woman is presenting in what appears to be a normal, established labour, and there are no signs of any complications at this point. The labour should be allowed to progress, and a repeat assessment should be performed at the interval specified by hospital guidelines (usually 2–4 hours).

 B

This patient is a multipara in established labour, with a deeply engaged fetal head. The CTG is abnormal, with recurrent late deceleration. The specificity of the CTG is low, and unless there are contraindications to fetal blood sampling, the fetal acid base balance should be ascertained by scalp blood sampling. This would give a more accurate measure of fetal compromise or otherwise. If it is impossible to perform a fetal blood sample, because of inadequate cervical dilation or the presence of contraindication, then immediate delivery by the speediest route is indicated.

 D

This patient has developed uterine hyperstimulation in response to vaginal prostaglandins, as evidenced by frequent contractions (seven in every 10 minutes) and the resulting CTG abnormalities. The first step in this woman's management would be to try and achieve uterine relaxation using a tocolytic; subcutaneous terbutaline would be the most appropriate option from the list. If there is no prompt response to tocolysis then delivery by Caesarean section should be the next step. It would be difficult to obtain a fetal scalp blood sample in the presence of an uneffaced, undilated cervix.

 F

Active management of the third stage of labour has been shown to reduce the risk of post-partum haemorrhage and the need for blood transfusion. It consists of administration of a uterotonic drug (usually ergometrin, oxytocin or a combination of both, syntometrin), early clamping of the cord and delivery of the placenta by controlled cord traction. The disadvantages are related predominantly to the drug effects, for example hypertension, headache, nausea and vomiting, and tachycardia.

Theme: Puerperal complications

 C

This patient is hypoxic, with tachypnoea and tachycardia, and a raised jugular venous pressure. There are no chest signs and she is apyrexial. Against the background of a high BMI, post-partum state and the history of emergency Caesarean section, pulmonary embolism has to be the main differential diagnosis. Venous thrombo-embolism is the leading cause of maternal mortality in the UK, and an active approach to investigation and treatment of women with suggestive symptoms and/or signs should be the norm.

 J

This patient's symptoms are compatible with overt psychosis. Puerperal psychosis can occur within the first week post-partum, and there may be serious risk to mother and baby. Symptoms can include mood abnormality, paranoid symptoms, delusions, hallucination and bizarre behaviour. Caesarean section is a risk factor, as are past history of psychosis, being unsupported and perinatal death. Puerperal psychosis constitutes a psychiatric emergency. Post-natal depression tends to occur later (peak onset in weeks 3–4) and the symptoms are usually those of depressive illness.

 D

The most likely cause of this patient's puerperal pyrexia is endometritis. This is supported by the physical signs of uterine tenderness and offensive lochia. Prolonged labour, failed instrumental delivery and emergency Caesarean section in labour are risk factors.

 B

This is a 'freebie' question! This woman has a UTI, as evidenced by the absence of a competing diagnosis and the findings on urinalysis.

G

Tenderness and redness over this woman's breast suggest mastitis. Breast abscess is not the best answer here, as the description clearly states the erythematous area to be 'non-fluctuant'. Mastitis can develop as a result of an infection (commonly staphylococcal) or as a result of a blocked milk duct; treatment is with a broad-spectrum penicillin. Continuation of breastfeeding is encouraged. A breast abscess can ensue if tissue necrosis occurs and a thick-walled, cystic area with pus develops – this can present as a tender breast mass. Treatment is by incision and drainage.

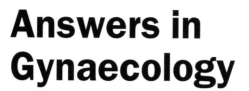

Answers in
Gynaecology

23

Anatomy and sexual differentiation

Theme: Pelvic anatomy

 I

The ovaries are attached to the uterus via the ovarian ligament. It is the most posterior structure to attach to the uterine cornu. It is followed, in anterior direction, by the fallopian tube, and then by the round ligament.

 A

As discussed in the previous answer, the structure anterior to the fallopian tube is the round ligament (*ligamentum teres uteri*).

 H

If the ovaries are being removed at hysterectomy, their connection to the pelvic sidewall has to be divided. This is the infundibulo-pelvic ligament (*ligamentum suspensorium ovarii*), *not* the ovarian ligament (*ligamentum ovarii proprium*), which, in turn, connects the ovary to the uterine cornu.

F

Endometriosis, which often presents with dysmenorrhoea and dyspareunia, commonly affects the uterosacral ligaments, which are situated behind the uterus. Their uterine insertion can be palpated through the posterior vaginal fornix during a bimanual vaginal examination.

(A115) D

Cervical carcinoma spreads, *per continuitatem*, laterally though the broad ligaments to the pelvic sidewall. More specifically, it would spread primarily via the transverse cervical ligaments (cardinal ligaments), which are situated in the caudal portion of the broad ligament.

Theme: Sexual differentiation and development

 D

This is a typical description of Klinefelter's syndrome, the most common chromosomal disorder associated with male hypogonadism. There are other karyotypic variants (XXXY, XXYY, etc.), but XXY is the most common pattern. Other features of Klinefelter's syndrome may include tall stature and small testes and penis, feminine fat distribution, and absent facial, axillary and pubic hair and low gonadotrophin levels.

(A117) B

This is Turner's syndrome. (See also 'Genetic disorders' in Chapter 2.)

 H

There are a number of endocrine conditions that prevent a genotypically normal male individual from developing a male phenotype (testicular feminisation, androgen insensitivity, 5-alpha-reductase deficiency). The common factor in most is that testosterone is unable to exert its effects. 5-Alpha-reductase deficiency is an autosomal recessive condition that results in the inability to convert testosterone into its physiologically more active form, dihydrotestosterone. In some individuals partial virilisation may occur at puberty because some isoenzymes increase in activity and may be able to engage testosterone receptors.

 A

An absent uterus is seen in Müllerian agenesis, which is an embryological rather than an endocrine problem. The Müllerian (paramesonephric) ducts give rise to uterus, fallopian tubes and the upper portion of the vagina. Ovaries are not affected, and the hormonal profile is therefore normal, with normal secondary sexual characteristics. The reason for seeking medical help is primarily amenorrhoea. Individuals with Müllerian agenesis usually have a normal female karyotype.

 A

This woman has *secondary* amenorrhoea, and she has had two pregnancies previously. Her karyotype is therefore likely to be 46 XX. Other causes of secondary amenorrhoea need to be sought.

24
Sexual health and family planning

Theme: Female genital tract infections

 B

The description of symptoms and signs in this case suggest genital herpes. Patients with a severe primary episode of genital herpes are often admitted with pain and may develop urinary retention.

 A

The patient in this case is likely to have acute PID, which is usually the result of an ascending, sexually transmitted infection. The history of ectopic pregnancy is relevant because of its association with chlamydial infection. The causative organism is *Chlamydia trachomatis*. The *C. psittaci* variety causes the influenza-like illness 'psittacosis'.

 G

Vulval warts result from an infection with the human papilloma virus, types 6 and 11. HPV Types 16 and 18, on the other hand, are associated with cervical cancer rather than warts.

A124 D

This history and microbiology suggest Group B streptococci (GBS), which are present in the vaginal flora of a substantial proportion of healthy women. The prevalence depends on the population make-up, generally between 15% and 30%. It is relevant in pregnancy because of the risk of fetal exposure during labour and delivery; intrapartum or neonatal infection can lead to severe neonatal sepsis. Screening for GBS is controversial, but intrapartum treatment is recommended. Carriers receive intravenous penicillin during labour to protect the fetus.

 A125 H

In the absence of barrier contraception, an irritant and offensive vaginal discharge suggests a sexually transmitted disease. The most likely organism from the option list to cause this type of discharge is *Trichomonas vaginalis*.

Theme: Family planning

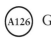 **A126** G

An IUCD is more appropriate in this case than Levonelle, because the patient has had a number of episodes of unprotected sexual intercourse during this cycle, as far as five days ago. The post-coital IUCD can be inserted up to five days after unprotected intercourse, but in reality it can be inserted up to five days after the earliest expected ovulation. In a stable 28-day cycle, the earliest expected ovulation is on day 14, which means that an IUCD could be inserted up to day 19 of the cycle. The IUCD will prevent up to 98% of expected pregnancies, compared to 95% prevented with Levonelle. Screening for STD under these circumstances should be the norm, as should advice regarding future contraception.

(A127) F

In the presence of heavy periods, the best choice for this patient would be the levonorgestrel intrauterine system (IUS). Apart from its contraceptive benefits, the device is highly successful in the treatment of heavy periods. Problems with weight gain are less common with the IUS than with injectable or subcutaneous progestogens.

(A128) B

The combined oral contraceptive pill is particularly suitable for this patient, because of its contraceptive efficacy as well as its non-contraceptive benefits. It is likely to improve her menstrual symptoms. However, advice on the use of additional barrier methods should be given, to protect her from STD.

(A129) J

The most useful method for this patient will be the implantable progestogen. It does not require repeated three-monthly access to the drug, and rare but possible problems that can be encountered with the levonorgestrel IUS, such as expulsion, will be avoided. Although amenorrhoea often ensues, there is a potential for un-scheduled vaginal bleeding with most progestogen-only methods, and access to sanitary protection may be required.

(A130) D

This patient with multiple medical problems, a stenosed cervical os and a reluctance to use contraceptive methods that would affect her menstrual pattern, is difficult to advise. The best option – provided she and her partner are in a stable relationship – is vasectomy.

25

Physiology and pathology of the menstrual cycle

Theme: Physiology of menstruation

 A

The post-ovulatory rise in core body temperature is mediated by the rise in progesterone secretion. It occurs in the early luteal phase following ovulation. The rise in temperature ranges between 0.5 °C and 1.0 °C. It is not entirely reliable because ovulation can occasionally take place without a demonstrable temperature rise.

 A

If ovulation occurs, the corpus luteum begins to secrete progesterone; a rise in plasma progesterone levels in the mid-luteal phase is therefore suggestive of an ovulatory cycle. In longer cycles the best timing for the test is one week before expected menstruation.

 E

Ovulation prediction kits for home use are based on the detection of the LH surge. Urine samples are tested during the presumed periovulatory period, usually for five consecutive days, so that intercourse can be timed accordingly. The usefulness of ovulation prediction kits is debatable. In patients whose cycles vary largely in duration (more than approximately a week), it may be difficult to pinpoint ovulation. The best advice usually is to have regular intercourse throughout the cycle.

B

Cyclical changes in the amount and consistency of cervical mucus form the basis for some natural family planning methods. As the proliferative phase progresses towards ovulation, rising oestrogen levels are associated with increasing amounts of clear cervical mucus, which is 'cohesive' (*spinnbarkeit*). In the luteal phase mucus becomes thicker, white and clumpy.

 A

The premenstrual-tension-type symptoms described in the case scenario are believed to be predominantly progesterone-induced; they are attributed to some progesterone metabolites such as allo-pregnanolone.

Theme: Histopathology of the endometrium

 E

Cyclical combined HRT is usually provided in 28-day packs; it is designed to emulate natural cycles as closely as possible. During the first 14 days of the pack the tablets/patches contain oestrogen only, followed by an oestrogen/progestogen combination for the latter 14 days. Under ideal circumstances the endometrial pattern would reflect this, i.e. in the in the first half of the pack endometrium would be proliferative, followed by secretory change in the second half.

 F

In analogy to miscarriage, tubal abortion implies that a tubal pregnancy has been spontaneously expelled from the fallopian tube. In pregnancy the endometrium is converted into decidua; as this is a hormonal effect, it occurs regardless of the implantation site. In the presence of an ectopic pregnancy, the uterine lining would typically be decidualised but there would be no evidence of trophoblast or embryonal tissue in the curettings.

(A138) C

The patient in this case scenario has no obvious risk factors for endometrial hyperplasia or malignancy, and there is no mention of HRT use. In the presence of thin endometrium (less than 5 mm) on transvaginal ultrasound it is therefore likely that the endometrium will be atrophic.

(A139) B

In contrast to the previous case, the patient portrayed here has many risk factors for endometrial carcinoma, including nulliparity, obesity, hypertension and diabetes. Her endometrial thickness is increased on transvaginal ultrasound (5 mm or more). The most likely histological finding therefore is adenocarcinoma. Hyperplasia is, of course, possible as a precursor; however, the constellation of risk factors characterises this patient as a candidate for cancer.

(A140) A

This patient, with moderately heavy and regular periods, is relatively unlikely to have significant endometrial pathology. As she is sterilised and there is no mention of exogenous hormones in the case scenario, we have to assume that we are looking at a natural cycle. Day 10 of the cycle would therefore fall into the proliferative phase, and that is what one would expect to see under the microscope.

Theme: Menstrual disorders

 C

The patient appears to have significant menstrual problems, resulting in anaemia and the need for iron therapy. The two main management principles in this case scenario are to treat the woman's symptoms and, as the woman is above the age of 40 and her cycles are irregular, to exclude an underlying malignancy. Baseline investigations should include a FBC and endometrial histology as a minimum. We already have the patient's recent Hb, so the next step would be an endometrial biopsy. In some centres an outpatient hysteroscopy might be performed at the same time. Pelvic ultrasound scan is less of a priority here because the pelvic examination is normal, although it might be useful if fibroids or other pelvic masses are suspected. Thyroid function tests are only performed if other symptoms of thyroid dysfunction are present.

 F

This patient has regular, heavy periods and endometrial pathology is therefore not very likely, although not impossible, particularly in obese women. The main issue in this case is that adequate pelvic assessment is impossible because of the patient's habitus. As there is marked adnexal tenderness, an ultrasound scan would be the most useful next step.

 A

This patient may have a pituitary microadenoma, which can give rise to hyperprolactinaemia and headaches. The visual disturbances typically seen with this condition would be the result of the compression of the *chiasma opticum*, which would result in visual field defects. The absence of visual field defects does not exclude a pituitary microadenoma. Other causes of raised prolactin levels include pregnancy and a number of drugs, including some antipsychotic medications, such as phenothiazines.

I

In women who have first-degree relatives with venous thrombo-embolism, thrombophilia screening should be considered prior to commencing the combined oral contraceptive pill. Familial thrombophilias include, amongst others, factor V Leiden mutation, protein C, S or antithrombin III deficiency and prothrombin mutations.

(A145) J

Post-coital and intermenstrual bleeding are symptoms that may be associated with cervical carcinoma. The patient's cervical screening history should be explored, and her cervix should be inspected. Occasionally a local cause will be found, such as a cervical polyp.

Theme: Amenorrhoea/ oligomenorrhoea

Although the table appears daunting at the first glance, you can answer this type of question comfortably by reading the case scenario and determining what the main feature of the endocrine profile would be in each case; you can then identify the option(s) with that particular feature and not be unnerved by the distractors!

 F

Secondary amenorrhoea with galactorrhoea is usually caused by a pregnancy or by hyperprolactinaemia of other aetiology. The endocrine profile to look for therefore would be one with markedly raised prolactin levels.

A

Secondary amenorrhoea associated with climacteric symptoms such as hot flushes and sweats, insomnia, forgetfulness, vaginal dryness and reduced libido, occurring in a woman in her mid-forties, is likely to be the menopause. The typical endocrine changes of the menopause include a marked rise in FSH and LH (hyper-gonadotrophic amenorrhoea).

 D

The amenorrhoea of severe weight loss, such as that associated with anorexia nervosa, is usually hypogonadotrophic in nature. The most likely endocrine profile therefore will be one with sub-stantially suppressed gonadotrophin levels.

 B

This case scenario is a good example of a patient presenting with polycystic ovarian syndrome. Other symptoms may include amenor-rhoea, hirsutism and infertility. Typically, there will be an inverse LH/FSH ratio (LH level three-fold the FSH level), low SHBG and raised free androgen index (the measure of testosterone unbound by SHBG). The option list contains only one option with a mark-edly inverse LH/FSH ratio!

 F

This is a variation on the presentation of hyperprolactinaemia; in this case a pituitary adenoma is likely to be responsible. Go for the one with high prolactin.

26
Infertility

Theme: Investigating infertile couples

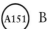 **B**

Whilst a number of investigations from the option list will be indicated, the single most useful investigation is going to be semen analysis. The partner's history of mumps raises the possibility of mumps epididymo-orchitis, which can result in male factor infertility.

A152 **A**

This patient is likely to have Asherman's syndrome. Intrauterine synaechiae (adhesions) develop as a result of vigorous curettage of the – usually post-partum – uterus, where the endometrium has been denuded. Similar synaechiae form following endometrial ablation in menstrual disorders, where this outcome is, in fact, intentional and therapeutic. The result is hypomenorrhoea, or light periods.

A153 **G**

This patient is likely to have tubal factor infertility following PID. Assessment would include an STD screen; however, this would not be accomplished by simply performing a high vaginal swab. The most useful investigation here in terms of infertility investigations would be to check tubal patency.

J

Whilst a number of investigations from the option list will be indicated, the most informative investigation here will be a serum prolactin level. Antipsychotic drugs, in particular phenothiazines, can lead to hyperprolactinaemia with resulting amenorrhoea/oligomenorrhoea and infertility.

 I

This patient is not, by definition, infertile, as she has not been trying to conceive for more than 12 months yet. There is clearly the need for education and reassurance here. However, all patients trying to conceive should be advised to take folic acid supplements and should have their rubella immunity checked. If they have no or low immunity, vaccination should be undertaken before pregnancy, and reliable contraception should be used for three months after the vaccine.

Theme: Causes of infertility

 A

The history of abdominal pain and abnormal vaginal discharge following IUCD insertion is suggestive of ascending genital infection; tubal damage and subsequent infertility can ensue.

 B

Primary infertility, dyspareunia and secondary dysmenorrhoea are characteristically present in endometriosis. Symptoms may be kept at bay for long periods by the use of the combined oral contraceptive pill, and are often exacerbated once the pill is discontinued.

C

The information given about the patient is rather scant, but it is clear that there is a high BMI and oligomenorrhoea. Under these circumstances the most likely cause for her failure to conceive is absent or infrequent ovulation, such as occurs with PCOS.

 H

The difficulty here appears to lie in the couple's lifestyle, with long intervals between episodes of sexual activity. There is nothing in the case scenario that would suggest any pathology.

 G

Antisperm antibodies can impair motility, lead to sperm clumping and may impair their ability to fertilise the egg. They are not particularly common in general, but may be detectable in up to 10% of infertile men. There is a strong association with male genital tract surgery; almost 70% of men who have undergone a vasectomy reversal will have antisperm antibodies. Women can develop antisperm antibodies, too; however, this is uncommon (less than 5% of infertile women).

27

Common gynaecological presentations

Theme: Urinary symptoms

 C

The constellation of symptoms including frequency and urgency, suggests a degree of detrusor instability. Caffeine intake is an associated factor, and after excluding a urinary tract infection, she would be advised in the first instance to reduce her coffee intake. Patients who fail to respond to first-line treatment should undergo a formal urodynamic assessment.

 B

This patient's symptoms are compatible with genuine stress incontinence (now termed 'urodynamic stress incontinence'). The frequency described in the case scenario is voluntary, resulting from the patient's anxiety about embarrassing incidents. Again, lifestyle issues such as weight loss and heavy lifting are addressed where appropriate, and pelvic floor exercises may be offered in the first instance. If first-line treatment is unsuccessful, the nature of the bladder dysfunction is confirmed by urodynamic assessment.

G

The symptoms described are compatible with a urinary tract infection. Occasionally, a ring pessary that is too large may compress the urethra against the pubic bone, resulting in a degree of voiding difficulty and residual urine in the bladder, which can then make the patient susceptible to infection. A severe voiding difficulty, leading to a large residual and overflow incontinence, is very rare. On the other hand, where the prolapse is large, correcting the position of the pelvic organs by a pessary or by surgery may sometimes reveal an underlying stress incontinence, which may have been obscured by a 'kinked' urethra associated with a complete procidentia.

 D

This patient clearly has urinary retention with overflow incontinence. The presentation following childbirth is characteristic: often, women have had a regional anaesthetic, prolonged labour and an instrumental delivery with resulting perineal trauma. All these factors predispose to urinary retention; this can go undiagnosed if small voiding volumes are ignored. If there is any concern about bladder function post-partum, a bladder scan can be performed to confirm complete bladder emptying; alternatively, a post-void catheterisation can be performed, although non-invasive techniques may be preferable.

 E

Protracted, obstructed labour can result in tissue necrosis in the vagina and surrounding tissues. Vesico-vaginal fistulae can ensue, and are commonly seen in the developing world where access to healthcare and obstetric services is poor.

Theme: Abnormal vaginal bleeding

 J

Anovulation is a common cause of irregular and heavy periods in adolescents. There is also an increase in the incidence of anovulatory cycles in perimenopausal women, so it is common in both extremes of the reproductive age spectrum.

 H

This patient has post-menopausal bleeding and her symptoms need to be investigated. However, with an endometrial thickness of <5 mm on transvaginal ultrasound, urogenital atrophy is the most likely cause. If her symptoms persist endometrial sampling should still be performed to exclude malignancy.

 A

The patient here is relatively young, with regular periods and no intermenstrual bleeding. There is no evidence of uterine enlargement/fibroids on pelvic examination. The most likely diagnosis therefore is dysfunctional uterine bleeding. Under these circumstances, first-line treatment can be administered without further investigation (apart from excluding anaemia). Additional tests need only be performed if there are symptoms or signs of co-morbidity (such as thyroid dysfunction) or if the patient fails to respond to first-line therapy.

 D

The symptoms of regular heavy periods and the presence of a large, irregular uterus suggest the diagnosis of fibroids. Additionally, the patient's ethnic origin places her in a group with a high prevalence of fibroids.

C

As discussed in the answer on endometrial histology earlier, a patient with the above characteristics is at high risk of endometrial carcinoma.

Theme: Pelvic pain

 I

The symptoms and findings in this case suggest endometriosis. The most useful investigation is diagnostic laparoscopy, which will help confirm or refute the suspected diagnosis; it will also help to rule out other differential diagnoses, such as PID.

 E

This patient has symptoms suggestive of STD, supported by her sexual history. She needs to be appropriately investigated to identify the micro-organism responsible. Additional measures would include antibiotic treatment for her and her partner and referral to genito-urinary medicine for follow-up and contact tracing.

 B

This patient clearly has a history of sub-fertility secondary to tubal disease. If she were to conceive, she would be at high risk of ectopic pregnancy. The first step here would be to do a pregnancy test; if this is positive, she would need to have an ultrasound scan to confirm the location of the pregnancy.

 F

As we know from the negative HCG result that the patient is not pregnant, the best option from the list is a pelvic ultrasound. Occasionally a persistent follicle can lead to a missed period and unilateral pelvic pain, and an ultrasound scan would help to confirm this diagnosis.

I

Ectopic pregnancy is very likely here. In a normal pregnancy, serum b-HCG should double every 48 hours. A sub-optimal rise (or fall) or the failure to visualise an intrauterine pregnancy on transvaginal ultrasound suggest an extrauterine pregnancy. A diagnostic laparoscopy is essential to establish a diagnosis.

28

Cancer in gynaecology

Theme: Treatment of female genital tract cancer

 A

Surgical treatment for carcinoma of the cervix is feasible until and including stage IIa. Radiotherapy is another option; however, ovarian function can be reliably preserved with surgery but not with radiotherapy. In younger women, preservation of ovarian function is clearly desirable and surgery may therefore be preferable unless there are other contraindications.

 J

This is stage III cervical carcinoma; it is too advanced for surgery, and radiotherapy is the first-line treatment.

 G

Stage IV ovarian carcinoma includes parenchymal liver metastases; the best mode of treatment is chemotherapy. Ovarian cancer is chemosensitive, and responds well to platinum-based and alkylating angents, and to taxoids.

D

In most patients, a well-differentiated adenocarcinoma can be treated by total abdominal hysterectomy and bilateral salpingo-oophorectomy. The need for adjuvant radiotherapy is largely determined by the depth of myometrial invasion and the grade of the tumour.

 E

This patient will require a radical vulvectomy, because of the size of the lesion and the presence of lymphadenopathy.

29

Screening and prevention

Theme: Women's health

 C

This patient has multiple risk factors for carcinoma of the cervix, including long-term use of the pill without barrier contraception, multiple sexual partners and smoking. Other risk factors include early age at first intercourse and HIV infection.

 H

A molar pregnancy can result in a choriocarcinoma. All patients with hydatidiform moles are followed up in specialist centres until six months after their beta-HCG levels become negative. They also need follow-up after every subsequent pregnancy, regardless of outcome.

 B

This patient has been exposed to unopposed oestrogen over a prolonged period of time. Whilst the absorption of topical oestrogens can be limited, it can amount to the endometrial hyperplasia/cancer threshold.

 F

This patient is at risk of developing breast cancer, because of the long-term use of combined HRT. The absolute increase in risk is small, but has been confirmed in a number of large studies. Combined HRT seems to be more of an issue in terms of breast cancer risk than oestrogen-only preparations.

I

Sub-fertility *per se* and ovulation induction treatment, in particular, have been linked to an increased risk of ovarian cancer.

Theme: Cervical screening

 E

This patient had an abnormal smear eight years ago, with normal smears since. Now that the cervix has been removed she can be discharged from the screening programme. However, in women with a recent cervical intraepithelial neoplasia (CIN) III, or where the cervix has been incompletely excised, it may be necessary to follow up with vaginal vault smears.

 E

Patients over the age of 65 who have always had normal smears can be discharged from the screening programme.

 C

Immediate referral for colposcopy is warranted in the presence of moderate or severe dyskaryosis, and abnormal glandular cells. Mild dyskaryosis warrants referral after two consecutive smears, and borderline smears after three occasions.

 B

An inadequate smear needs to be repeated to obtain a usable slide that can be read.

 C

After three borderline smears colposcopy is required.

30
Operative gynaecology

Theme: Peri-operative complications

 F

The main objective of surgical management of ovarian cancer is debulking (reducing tumour mass), which can involve extensive surgery, and bowel involvement in the tumour is not uncommon. Complications such as paralytic ileus and bowel obstruction can ensue. In this case, nausea and vomiting, together with a distended abdomen, suggest a bowel complication; as bowel sounds are absent, paralytic ileus is likely.

 I

There are a number of differential diagnoses here that need to be considered, including pulmonary embolism. However, the clue lies in the statement that the patient's pain is poorly controlled, which, after a laparotomy, may lead to inadequate inspiration/chest expansion, and may result in hypoventilation of the lung bases and subsequent collapse of the affected lobes. Reduced air entry over the lung bases is typical of extensive atelectasis.

 A

This patient is likely to have a pulmonary embolus. Atelectasis in a fully mobile, well patient with good pain control is not likely, and there are no clues in the case scenario that would lead to a competing diagnosis. Tachycardia is a significant finding here, it is often present in pulmonary embolism.

C

Uterine perforation, particularly in a pregnant uterus, is a serious complication. It can lead to substantial haemorrhage requiring a hysterectomy, but also other organs such as bowel can be injured, in particular where a suction curette is being used for the uterine evacuation. Typical clues would be difficult dilation of the cervix, failure to obtain tissues on curettage and insertion of the curette to a depth beyond the expected size of the uterine cavity. Laparoscopy/laparotomy to inspect the damage and deal with any injuries is required.

 D

Serious injury to bowel or blood vessels (aorta, vena cava) occurs in approximately 1:2000–3000 laparoscopies. Whilst injury to major vessels usually becomes symptomatic very quickly, bowel injury may not be detected until faecal peritonitis develops several days later.

Theme: Surgical management in gynaecology

 I

Ruptured ectopic pregnancy is a life-threatening gynaecological emergency. Minimal access surgery is not appropriate in this case scenario, and a laparotomy and salpingectomy should be performed without delay.

 H

A persistent or symptomatic simple cyst in a young patient, where there is low likelihood of malignancy, can be dealt with via minimal access surgery. Options include a laparoscopic cystectomy, where some ovarian tissue is preserved, and oophorectomy, where the entire ovary is removed. The size of the cyst and amount of residual healthy ovarian tissue will determine which of the two is more feasible. Cyst aspiration is not considered an adequate alternative because of the high recurrence rate (50%); however, the cyst can also be fenestrated (de-roofed).

 E

Several items in the case scenario indicate a high risk of malignancy: the patient is post-menopausal, the cysts are complex and they are bilateral. Whilst the CA 125 level is normal in this patient, it is only raised in about 80% of ovarian cancers, and should only be seen in the context of history and other findings. Almost half of post-menopausal women undergoing an operation for an ovarian mass will have cancer.

 G

An unruptured ectopic pregnancy in a stable patient is amenable to minimal access surgery. This patient can be treated by laparoscopic salpingectomy.

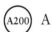 **A**

A vaginal hysterectomy would not be appropriate in a patient with large fibroids, and at the age of 30 years oophorectomy would not be appropriate in the presence of normal ovaries. A sub-total hysterectomy is therefore the best option from the list, although a total abdominal hysterectomy could also be performed. Whilst there have been multiple failed attempts at conservative management of menorrhagia, surgery remains a difficult option in a patient who will not accept blood transfusion. If surgery is embarked on, attempts should be made to bring her pre-operative haemoglobin into a normal range, perhaps by inducing amenorrhoea with GnRH analogues. Intraoperative blood loss should be minimised and a sub-total hysterectomy, where the cervix is left *in situ*, leads to a shorter operating time and less blood loss than total hysterectomy. This option should only be considered if the patient's smear history is unremarkable.

Theme: Devices and instruments in gynaecology

 A

NICE guidelines suggest that Filshie clips or Falope rings should be used as a method of tubal occlusion rather than diathermy. The devices are applied laparoscopically, so patients have to be made aware of potential operative risks.

 E

In post-menopausal women the squamo-columnar junction (SCJ) usually retracts into the endocervical canal. A cytobrush is used to access the SCJ and sample the transformation zone adequately. In women on HRT, who have a higher level of oestrogenation, the SCJ may be visible on the ectocervix. The Ayers spatula (option C) is also pictured; however, with the introduction of Liquid Based Cytology, it will be replaced by a broom-like device.

 J

A ring pessary is a vaginal device used for the conservative management of prolapse. Other types of pessaries are available, but less widely used.

 F

The assessment of the anterior vaginal wall is best performed with the patient in the Sim position (similar to recovery position), using a Sim speculum to retract the posterior vaginal wall and allow the inspection of the anterior vaginal wall. It was originally devised to help visualise vesico-vaginal fistulae.

 B

A uterine sound is used to measure the length of the uterine cavity prior to procedures such as curettage, endometrial ablation or insertion of intrauterine devices.

31
Therapeutics in gynaecology

Theme: Drug therapy in gynaecology

 A

Metronidazole is the appropriate treatment for *Trichomonas vaginalis* and for bacterial vaginosis, whilst doxycycline is effective in chlamydial infections.

 H

Detrusor contractions are initiated by the parasympathetic nervous system via the pelvic nerve; acetylcholine is released at the neuromuscular junction and a contraction ensues. Detrusor instability, therefore, responds well to anticholinergic medication, which blocks acetylcholine receptors. However, most anticholinergic drugs produce side effects such as dry mouth, drowsiness, tachycardia and visual disturbances, and this may affect compliance.

 J

In this case, metformin rather than Dianette is indicated because the patient wishes to conceive. Ovulation induction with clomiphene citrate may be necessary; there is some evidence that this is more successful if used in conjunction with metformin. However, it is important to bear in mind that metformin is used 'off label' under these circumstances, as it is only licensed for use in diabetes.

D

This is another case of PCOS, but here fertility is not currently an issue. As hirsutism is one of the presenting problems, a drug with anti-androgenic activity is likely to be appropriate; Dianette is therefore a good choice here. The combined oral contraceptive pill (COCP) will increase SHBG levels. Metformin is occasionally used under these circumstances, but its effectiveness in treating androgenic manifestations of PCOS is yet to be proven.

 I

Prolactin secretion is not suppressed by negative feedback from peripheral hormones; a short-loop feedback is in place, via the hypophyseal portal system and hypothalamic dopamine. A compression of the pituitary stalk will therefore disrupt the feedback mechanism and prolactin secretion will escape inhibition. Dopamine agonists such as bromocriptine and cabergoline are used in the pharmacological treatment of hyperprolactinaemia.

32
Ethics in obstetrics and gynaecology

Theme: Medico-legal and ethical principles 1

 B

When providing contraception for under-16s, it is important to establish whether they are competent under the Fraser Guidelines (so-called 'Gillick Competence') to make decisions about their treatment, or whether a parent or guardian needs to be notified. In adherence to the guidance, the healthcare professional treating the patient needs to establish and document the following:

- That the young person understands the practitioner's advice.
- That the young person cannot be persuaded to inform his or her parents or allow the practitioner to inform the parents that contraceptive advice has been sought.
- That the young person is likely to begin or to continue having intercourse with or without contraceptive treatment, and unless he or she receives contraceptive advice or treatment, the young person's physical or mental health is likely to suffer.
- The young person's best interest requires the practitioner to give contraceptive advice, treatment or both without parental consent.

The principle of confidentiality is also relevant here, but is largely influenced by the Gillick competence of the young person.

H

The procedure here was performed against the patient's express wishes. She declined an instrumental delivery; whilst it appears that she was in pain and distress, this does not make her, in legal terms, incompetent to decide on her medical treatment. Next of kin cannot give consent on behalf of a competent person, and certainly cannot override their refusal or consent. The healthcare professionals involved in this case have made themselves vulnerable to a charge of battery.

 D

There is a clear delay here in the response to the midwife's concerns by medical staff. If there is concern about fetal well-being, this has to be addressed in a speedy manner to avoid complications caused by asphyxia. Failure of medical staff to respond to the problem at hand is likely to be seen as negligence on their part.

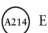 E

This case scenario is set out to describe a situation where a number of treatment options are available; however, the patient appears not to have been consulted about here wishes or preferences. The doctor has made the decision to proceed with surgery on her behalf; this suggests a paternalistic approach. Whilst there may be patients who express the wish to be guided by their doctor, a dialogue with the patients is always essential to enable them to make the choices appropriate for them. This patient may not have been given enough information about treatment alternatives to be able to give informed consent to the operation.

 A

Confidentiality is an important ethical principle governing the doctor–patient relationship. Under these circumstances, it may be in the patient's interest for the doctor to respond to the insurance queries and supply the relevant information; however, she still has to authorise the release of information to a third party.

Theme: Medico-legal and ethical principles 2

 G

Here, the family is asking you to withhold information from the patient, so strictly speaking they are not asking you to breach confidentiality. However, the ethical principle of veracity, being truthful with your patient, is the principle you are likely to disregard if you concede to the family's request. Whilst the family usually acts out of concern for the patient, it is entirely inappropriate to keep patients in the dark about their condition or treatment; the patient may specifically request not to be given particular details, but that is not the situation here. Interestingly, in some parts of the world it is seen as the correct approach and is, in fact, a cultural dictum to keep potentially 'harmful' information from the patient.

 A

In this case scenario you are, in fact, being asked to breach confidentiality. It is the patient who decides whether and what the family can be told about his or her condition, and not vice versa.

 F

Competent patients have the right to decide what should happen to them in terms of acceptance or refusal of medical treatment, even if the consequences of their decision are fatal. That right is enshrined in the principle of autonomy. The doctor's role is to give the patient appropriate information about treatment alternatives and management strategies that may be acceptable to him or her. Where there are concerns about the motivation for a particular decision, the patient's reasons for his or her choices should be explored and further information and support offered where appropriate.

B

The fact that the patient has a legal guardian suggests that she is not thought to be competent to make decisions such as consent to medical treatment. In an emergency situation, where the patient's life is at risk, doctors may act under the beneficence principle; however, the scenario suggests there is scope to await the arrival of the legal guardian.

 I

Doctors may act in the patient's best interest when informed consent is not obtainable (e.g. unconscious patient following an RTA, etc.) in situations where there is risk of significant harm or death, and the patient has not previously made a medical directive regarding refusal of particular interventions.